PUBLIC HEALTH IN THE 21ST CENTURY

ISSUES IN PROVIDING EMERGENCY MEDICAL CARE

PUBLIC HEALTH IN THE 21ST CENTURY

Additional books in this series can be found on Nova's website under the Series tab.

Additional E-books in this series can be found on Nova's website under the E-book tab.

PUBLIC HEALTH IN THE 21ST CENTURY

ISSUES IN PROVIDING EMERGENCY MEDICAL CARE

MARY E. MATHERS
EDITOR

Nova Science Publishers, Inc.
New York

For permission to use material from this book please contact us:
Telephone 631-231-7269; Fax 631-231-8175
Web Site: http://www.novapublishers.com

LIBRARY OF CONGRESS CATALOGING-IN-PUBLICATION DATA

Issues in providing emergency medical care / editor, Mary E. Mathers.
p. ; cm.
Includes index.
ISBN 978-1-61761-595-5 (hardcover)
1. Emergency medical services--United States. I. Mathers, Mary E.
[DNLM: 1. Emergency Medical Services. 2. Emergency Medical Services--economics. 3. Health Services Accessibility. WX 215]
RA645.5.I87 2010
362.18--dc22

2010031745

Published by Nova Science Publishers, Inc. † New York

CONTENTS

PREFACE

Hospital emergency departments are a major part of the nation's health care safety net. Of the estimated 119 million visits to U.S. emergency departments in 2006, over 40 percent were paid for by federally-supported programs. These programs, Medicare, Medicaid, and the State Children's Health Insurance Program, are administered by the Department of Health and Human Services (HHS). There have been reports of crowded conditions in emergency departments, often associated with adverse effects on patient quality of care. This book explores the issues in providing emergency medical care, including crowding in emergency hospital departments; emergency response and volunteer health professionals; ambulance providers; and public health and medical preparedness response

Chapter 1- The Emergency Medical Treatment and Active Labor Act (EMTALA) ensures universal access to emergency medical care at all Medicare participating hospitals with emergency departments. Under EMTALA, any person who seeks emergency medical care at a covered facility, regardless of ability to pay, immigration status, or any other characteristic, is guaranteed an appropriate screening exam and stabilization treatment before transfer or discharge. Failure to abide by these requirements can subject hospitals or physicians to civil monetary sanctions or exclusion from Medicare. Hospitals may also be subject to civil liability under the statute for personal injuries resulting from the violation

Chapter 2- Hospital emergency departments are a major part of the nation's health care safety net. Of the estimated 119 million visits to U.S. emergency departments in 2006, over 40 percent were paid for by federally-supported programs. These programs—Medicare, Medicaid, and the State Children's Health Insurance Program—are administered by the Department of

Health and Human Services (HHS). There have been reports of crowded conditions in emergency departments, often associated with adverse effects on patient quality of care. In 2003, GAO reported that most emergency departments in metropolitan areas experienced some degree of crowding (*Hospital Emergency Departments: Crowded Conditions Vary among Hospitals and Communities*, GAO-03-460). For example, two out of every three metropolitan hospitals reported going on ambulance diversion—asking ambulances to bypass their emergency departments and instead transport patients to other facilities.

GAO was asked to examine information made available since 2003 on emergency department crowding. GAO examined three indicators of emergency department crowding—ambulance diversion, wait times, and patient boarding—and factors that contribute to crowding. To conduct this work, GAO reviewed national data; conducted a literature review of 197 articles; and interviewed officials from HHS and professional and research organizations, and individual subject-matter experts.

Chapter 3- The devastation inflicted on the Gulf region by Hurricanes Katrina and Rita in 2005 and Hurricanes Gustav and Ike in 2008, in addition to recent disasters in the Midwest due to tornadoes and flooding, triggered mass relief efforts by local, state, and federal government agencies, as well as private organizations and individuals. As unpaid volunteers have carried out much of the relief effort, some have questioned whether such volunteers—particularly medical personnel, so-called "volunteer health professionals" (VHPs)—will be protected from potential civil liability in carrying out their duties. This chapter provides a general overview of the various federal and state liability protections available to VHPs responding to disasters. This chapter does not discuss liability of VHPs who go abroad to render assistance.

Chapter 4- Key recent events—the 2001 terrorist attacks, Hurricane Katrina, and concerns about an influenza ("flu") pandemic, among others—sharpened congressional interest in the nation's systems to track and respond to public health threats. The 109th Congress passed several laws that established, reorganized, or reauthorized key public health and medical preparedness and response programs in the Departments of Health and Human Services (HHS) and Homeland Security (DHS). The 110th Congress was engaged in oversight of the implementation of these laws, focused in particular on such matters as (1) the fitness of HHS and DHS—in terms of authority, funding, policies, and workforce—to respond to health emergencies; (2) the effectiveness of coordination among them and other federal agencies; and (3) the status of major initiatives such as pandemic flu preparedness and disaster planning for at-risk populations. The 111th Congress is likely to remain engaged in oversight of the nation's readiness for health threats.

The Obama Administration may reconsider homeland security objectives and priorities established by the George W. Bush Administration. Shifts in doctrine or priority, if any, may manifest as key positions are filled, or in the budget proposal for FY2010.

The 111th Congress may review HHS's disaster response capabilities, including its authority to declare a public health emergency and the means to fund its response efforts. Among other things, it is not clear that a flu pandemic would qualify for major disaster assistance under the Robert T. Stafford Disaster Relief and Emergency Assistance Act (the Stafford Act). Also, although the HHS Secretary has authority for a no-year Public Health Emergency Fund, Congress has not appropriated monies to the fund for many years. Finally, since Hurricane Katrina, Congress has urged and HHS has adopted a more aggressive federal role in the response to health emergencies

Chapter 5- In 2002, Medicare implemented a national fee schedule designed to standardize payments for ambulance services. The Medicare Prescription Drug, Improvement and Modernization Act of 2003 (MMA) required GAO to study ambulance service costs. GAO examined providers' costs of ground ambulance transports in 2004 and factors that contributed to cost differences; average Medicare ambulance payments expected under the national fee schedule in 2010 and how those payments will relate to providers' costs per transport; and changes that occurred in Medicare beneficiaries' use of ambulance transports from 2001 to 2004. GAO estimated costs of ambulance transports based on a nationally representative survey of 215 ambulance providers that did not share costs with nonambulance services. Providers that shared costs with other institutions or services and could not report their costs for ambulance services separately, such as fire departments, were excluded because their reported costs appeared unreliable. GAO used its survey, Medicare claims, and other data for its analyses.

In: Issues in Providing Emergency Medical Care ISBN: 978-1-61761-595-5
Editor: Mary E. Mathers

Chapter 1

EMTALA: ACCESS TO EMERGENCY MEDICAL CARE

Edward C. Liu

SUMMARY

The Emergency Medical Treatment and Active Labor Act (EMTALA) ensures universal access to emergency medical care at all Medicare participating hospitals with emergency departments. Under EMTALA, any person who seeks emergency medical care at a covered facility, regardless of ability to pay, immigration status, or any other characteristic, is guaranteed an appropriate screening exam and stabilization treatment before transfer or discharge. Failure to abide by these requirements can subject hospitals or physicians to civil monetary sanctions or exclusion from Medicare. Hospitals may also be subject to civil liability under the statute for personal injuries resulting from the violation.

OVERVIEW

In 1986, Congress enacted the Emergency Medical Treatment and Active Labor Act (EMTALA)[1] to address the problem of "patient dumping" in hospital emergency departments. Patient dumping refers to instances in which a hospital turns away indigent or uninsured persons seeking treatment so that the hospital will not have to absorb the cost of treating them. Although attempts to facilitate indigent access to emergency health care already existed in state and federal law, legal frameworks prior to EMTALA were plagued with poor enforcement mechanisms and vague standards of conduct.[2] Amid graphic media reports of hospitals sending away critically ill patients without proper stabilization treatment and delivery rooms unwilling to accept indigent or uninsured women in labor, Congress passed EMTALA as part of the Consolidated Omnibus Budget Reconciliation Act of 1985.[3]

EMTALA's statutory scheme has traditionally been deconstructed into two principal categories: (1) provisions that ensure an appropriate medical screening, and (2) provisions that require stabilization before transfer or discharge.[4] EMTALA only requires stabilization of whatever emergency conditions a hospital detects, and does not provide a right to indefinite care for anyone who comes to an emergency room. EMTALA's requirements may be suspended by the Secretary of Health and Human Services during national emergencies, such as the recent landfall of Hurricane Ike in Texas.[5] Hospitals and physicians that fail to comply with these requirements may be fined $50,000 and/or excluded from participation in Medicare, and hospitals may also be held civilly liable to persons who suffer personal injury.[6]

The Screening Requirement

Only hospitals that (1) participate in Medicare and (2) maintain an emergency department are required to screen patients under EMTALA.[7] Hospitals that do not have a "dedicated emergency department" are not subject to the screening requirement of EMTALA.[8] Similarly, emergency care providers that are unaffiliated with a hospital need not comply with EMTALA, even where those providers are the only medical care facilities reasonably accessible.[9] For example, in *Rodriguez v. American Int'l Ins. Co. of Puerto Rico*, the First Circuit declined to extend EMTALA protections to a 24-hour emergency room clinic in rural Puerto Rico because the clinic was not associated with a hospital. The Federal District Court for the District of Puerto Rico had initially held that, because the clinic was the primary provider of 24-hour emergency health care in its area, applying EMTALA to the clinic best furthered the statutory goal of universal access to emergency medical care.[10]

However, the First Circuit reversed, holding that any considerations of the goals of Congress were inappropriate where the text of the statute was clear.[11]

When is the Screening Requirement Triggered?

The screening requirement is triggered when an individual "comes to the emergency department" of a hospital and requests to be treated. [12] Under HHS regulations, an individual may be deemed to have come to the emergency department in certain circumstances, even though the individual is not physically present in the emergency department or elsewhere on the hospital campus.[13] For example, a patient en-route to a hospital in an ambulance or air transport owned by that hospital has "come to the emergency department" of that hospital and may not be refused a screening exam under EMTALA. These regulations also state that incoming patients in ambulances that are not owned by the receiving hospital have not "come to the emergency department." The regulations further allow the hospital to redirect the non-owned ambulance if the hospital is in "diversionary status."[14] However, at least one Federal Court of Appeal has rejected this interpretation of the statute and has held that EMTALA could be triggered by an incoming ambulance that was not owned by the receiving hospital.[15]

In *Morales v. Sociedad Espanola*, the hospital had argued that HHS regulations clearly state that patients in non-owned ambulances have not yet "come to the emergency department," and therefore EMTALA did not apply. However, according to the First Circuit's reading of the pertinent regulations, a hospital is only permitted to take the *affirmative action* of refusing a non-owned ambulances if it is actually in "diversionary status." The court argued that this reading gives effect to every word in the regulation and also best effectuates EMTALA's statutory goal of preventing patient dumping.[16]

Regardless of whether the ambulance is owned by a hospital or not, should an ambulance ignore a redirection request, EMTALA is triggered if the patient physically arrives on the hospital's property.[17]

What Constitutes an "Appropriate Screening Exam?"

Although hospitals with dedicated emergency departments are required to perform screening exams, it is not necessarily a violation of EMTALA if a screening exam falls short of either a local or national medical malpractice standard.[18] The language of the statute requires only "an appropriate medical screening exam."[19] The majority of the federal circuits have held that, because the chief evil sought to be prevented was the lack of access for uninsured patients, an "appropriate" exam is one comparable to what a paying patient would receive under similar circumstances.[20] However, the Sixth Circuit has construed the statute more narrowly, holding that there is no violation of EMTALA without the additional allegation of an "improper motive" that led to a substandard screening exam.[21]

THE STABILIZATION REQUIREMENT

Like the screening requirement, the stabilization requirement applies to all Medicare participating hospitals with a dedicated emergency department. However, in some cases the stabilization requirement may also apply to a Medicare participating hospital even if it does not have an emergency department. For example, if treatment of an individual's medical condition requires a particular hospital's unique equipment or expertise, federal regulations compel that hospital to accept a transfer of that patient from any nearby U.S. hospital.[22]

The stabilization requirement is triggered when a hospital discovers that an individual has an emergency medical condition. Actual knowledge of an emergency medical condition is required.[23] Therefore, if a hospital fails to accurately detect an individual's emergency condition and discharges that individual without stabilizing the medical condition, the hospital may not have violated EMTALA's stabilization provisions. However, the hospital may still be civilly liable to the individual based upon state medical malpractice claims if the failure to detect an emergency condition was due to negligence during the screening exam.[24]

Interpretations of the Stabilization Requirement

Except where medically necessary, hospitals must ensure that an individual is stabilized before discharge or transfer. Federal regulations define an individual as stabilized as either (1) when there is a reasonable assurance that no material deterioration would result from that individual's transfer or discharge from the hospital or, (2) in the case of women in labor, after delivery of the child and placenta.[25] Unlike the screening requirement, the language of the stabilization requirement does not qualify the care to be given as "appropriate."[26] Based on this textual distinction, the U.S. Supreme Court has held that no "improper motive" need be alleged to show a violation of EMTALA's stabilization provisions.[27]

Stabilization and inpatient status

When an emergency medical condition is detected, a hospital may decide to admit the individual as an inpatient for further treatment. Whether the stabilization requirement continues to apply to patients after they have been admitted is a disputed issue. Because the statute only defines "stabilization" in the context of transfers, the Fourth, Ninth and Eleventh Circuits have held that a hospital has no stabilization duties that are enforceable under EMTALA once an individual has been admitted.[28] However, the Sixth Circuit disagreed in *Thornton v. Southwest Detroit Hospital.*[29] In that case, a stroke victim alleged she was discharged from the ICU without being stabilized, in violation of EMTALA, after 21 days of inpatient care. The Sixth Circuit held that EMTALA still required stabilization before discharge, despite her inpatient status.[30]

The Supreme Court declined to rule on this issue in *Roberts v. Galen*, although it had an opportunity to do so.[31] However, during oral arguments for that case, an Assistant Solicitor General, arguing as amicus curiae, informed the Court that the Department of Health and Human Services intended to begin rule-making procedures to provide guidance on this question.[32] In 2002, the Centers for Medicare and Medicaid Services (CMS) issued a notice of a proposed rule extending EMTALA protections to inpatients.[33] Many solicited comments pointed to the *Bryant v. Adventist*[34] decision holding otherwise,[35] and in 2003, CMS reversed its position, stating that if, after performing a screening exam, a hospital admits an individual for treatment of an emergency medical condition, then the hospital has satisfied its duties under EMTALA.[36]

In August of 2008, HHS further clarified its position by stating that EMTALA does not apply to an individual who has been screened and admitted at one hospital but requires a transfer to a second hospital that has specialized facilities.[37] As described above, where a patient has not yet been admitted, nearby specialized hospitals are generally required to accept transfers of the patient from the original hospital.[38] However, the new regulations clearly state that once the individual has been admitted as an inpatient in one hospital, other specialized hospitals do not continue to have a duty to accept a transfer under EMTALA.[39]

Despite the promulgation of these rules, the Sixth Circuit has continued to hold that the mere admission of an individual, without further treatment, does not satisfy EMTALA.[40] The court in this case found the CMS regulations to be contrary to the plain language of the statute. Therefore, the regulations were inapplicable.[41] In particular, the court relied upon language in EMTALA which prohibits hospitals from releasing patients with emergency medical conditions without providing treatment to stabilize the condition. According to the court, the CMS regulations would permit hospitals to avoid EMTALA liability by simply admitting and immediately discharging patients, without providing any treatment. The court found such a construction to be unreasonable and contrary to the language of the statute.[42] However, one could argue that by admitting an individual, a hospital opens itself up to traditional medical malpractice liability under state law. Therefore, while the CMS regulations may provide a means of avoiding EMTALA liability by admitting and discharging individuals, compliance with EMTALA would not necessarily immunize hospitals from applicable state law claims. Insofar as the intent of EMTALA was to prevent situations in which hospitals could "dump" patients without incurring any liability, providing an incentive for hospitals to admit emergency room patients may be consistent with that goal. Once a patient is admitted, it could be argued that EMTALA liability is unnecessary as state medical malpractice law could provide an incentive for the hospital to ensure the provision of necessary stabilizing treatment.

Stabilization of known emergency conditions

The stabilization requirement may preempt certain state laws authorizing physicians to decline administering treatment where deemed inappropriate based upon their medical judgment. In In re Baby K, a hospital sought a declaratory judgment that they were permitted to refuse to treat an anencephalic infant in respiratory distress.[43] The hospital argued that the prevailing standard of care for anencephalic infants was to provide warmth and nutrition without mechanical respiration, and that Virginia state law authorized physicians to refuse to provide care they believed would be inappropriate.[44] The Fourth Circuit disagreed and held that the requirement of stabilization prior to transfer or discharge was compulsory once an emergency medical condition had been identified by hospital personnel, even where the treating physician believed stabilization treatment would have been futile. Furthermore, the court held that EMTALA preempted the Virginia statute authorizing the physician to refuse to provide treatment he reasonably believed to be inappropriate.[45]

Requirements for transfers after stabilization. All transfers must be conducted with qualified personnel and equipment. An individual may not be transferred unless the receiving hospital consents to receive the individual. The receiving hospital must have the capacity and expertise to treat the transferred individual, and all medical records must be sent to the receiving hospital. It is the transferring hospital's obligation to ensure that the transfer has been performed as described above and the transferring hospital remains liable under EMTALA until an appropriate transfer is completed.[46] It is not a violation of EMTALA to transfer an individual who has not been stabilized when it is medically necessary to do so. In such situations, a qualified medical person, as defined by the hospital's own rules and regulations, must certify that the benefits of transfer to a different facility outweigh the risks involved.[47]

Hospital Liability to Third Parties

EMTALA provides a civil remedy to "any individual who suffers personal harm as a direct result of a participating hospital's violation." In 2009, the Sixth Circuit held that this language provided a civil remedy to third parties that were injured as a direct result of a violation of either the screening or stabilization requirements.[48] In the case before the court, the hospital was alleged to have improperly discharged an emergency room patient who was psychiatrically unstable. Ten days after his discharge the patient murdered his wife. The wife's estate subsequently brought suit against the hospital alleging that the hospital's failure to stabilize before discharge was a direct cause of her death. The defendants argued that the patient's wife lacked standing under EMTALA because it only permitted civil claims by persons that were personally denied treatment in violation of the statute. In support of this argument, the defendants noted that, during consideration of EMTALA, the House Judiciary Committee had issued a report stating

> [The civil suit provision of EMTALA] authorizes only two types of actions for damages. The first of these could be brought by the individual patient who suffers harm as a direct result of [a] hospital's failure to appropriately screen, stabilize, or properly transfer that patient. The second type of action could be brought by a medical facility which received an improperly transferred emergency patient.[49]

Because third parties were not mentioned in the legislative history, the defendants argued that this suit should not be permitted. The Sixth Circuit disagreed, noting that

> where a House committee's explanation of the meaning of a statute seems to differ from the statute's actual wording, this Court should not rely on that committee's statement as the exclusive explanation for the meaning of the statute.... We recognize that our interpretation of the civil enforcement provision may have consequences for hospitals that Congress may or may not have considered or intended. However, our duty is only to read the statute as it is written.[50]

In the court's view, the statutory text afforded a civil remedy to "*any* individual who suffers personal harm as a direct result" of the hospital's actions, and the most logical reading of this text permits suits to be brought by harmed third parties.[51]

End Notes

[1] P.L. 99-272, 100 Stat. 164 (1986) codified at 42 U.S.C. § 1395dd et seq. (2007).

[2] Tiana Mayere Lee, *An EMTALA Primer: The Impact of Changes in the Emergency Medicine Landscape on EMTALA Compliance and Enforcement*, 13 ANNALS OF HEALTH L. 145, 146-147 (2004) (discussing the Hill-Burton Act and state statutory and common law). *See also* H.Rept. 99-241, pt. 3, at 5 (1985) (discussing state remedies).

[3] Lee, *supra* note 2 at 147-148, 151.

[4] 42 U.S.C. § 1395dd(a), (b).

[5] 42 U.S.C. § 1320b-5(b)(3). *See* Waiver or Modification of Requirements Under Section 1135 of the Social Security Act, Michael O. Leavitt, Secretary of the Department of Health and Human Services, (Sept. 11, 2008), *available at* http://www.hhs.gov/disasters/emergency/naturaldisasters/hurricanes. Sanctions are only lifted for inappropriate transfers or redirections. 42 C.F.R. § 489.24(a)(2).

[6] 42 U.S.C. § 1395dd(d). Civil fines are limited to $25,000 for hospitals with fewer than 100 beds. *Id.* at (d)(1)(A). Private suits may not be brought against physicians individually. *See e.g. Heimlicher v. Steele*, 442 F. Supp. 2d 685 (N.D. Iowa 2006) (citing *King v. Ahrens*, 16 F.3d 265 (8th Cir. 1994), *Delaney v. Cade*, 986 F.2d 387 (10th Cir. 1993), and *Baber v. Hosp. Corp. of Am.*, 977 F.2d 872 (4th Cir. 1992)). Medicare termination appears to be infrequently invoked as a sanction. Laura D. Hermer, *The Scapegoat: EMTALA and Emergency Department Overcrowding*, 14 J. L. & Policy 695, 701 n. 29 (2006) (stating that between 1986 and 2001 only four hospitals had their Medicare agreements terminated).

[7] 42 U.S.C. § 1395dd(a), (d)(1)(A), and (e)(2). Although the screening and stabilization requirements are phrased such that they apply to "hospitals" generally, enforcement of EMTALA is only authorized against hospitals that have entered into a Medicare provider agreement. *Id.*

[8] 42 U.S.C. § 1395dd(a). A dedicated emergency department is defined as any facility that is licensed or held out to the public as such, or that provides urgent care to one third of its outpatients during the preceding calendar year. 42 C.F.R. § 489.24(b).

[9] *Rodriguez v. American Int'l Ins. Co. of Puerto Rico*, 402 F.3d 45 (1st Cir. 2005).

[10] *Rodriguez v. American Int'l Ins. Co. of Puerto Rico*, 263 F. Supp. 2d 297 (D. Puerto Rico 2003) (arguing that the nature of the services provided should be determinative, not whether a facility is defined as a hospital).

[11] *Rodriguez v. American Int'l*, 402 F.3d at 49 (noting that Congress was free in drafting the statute to extend EMTALA to rural clinics unaffiliated with hospitals, but had not done so). EMTALA does apply to facilities designated as "critical access hospitals," which provide 24-hour emergency services and acute inpatient care to rural areas. 42 U.S.C. § 1395dd(e)(5).

[12] 42 U.S.C. § 1395dd(a). Requests for treatment may be made on the individual's behalf and a request may be implied if a prudent layperson observer would believe that the individual needs emergency medical care. 42 C.F.R. § 489.24(b) (2006).

[13] 42 C.F.R. § 489.24(b). The campus includes areas within 250 yards of a hospital's main buildings. 42 C.F.R. § 413.65(b).

[14] 42 C.F.R. § 489.24(b). A hospital is in diversionary status if it lacks the staff or facilities to treat additional emergency patients. *See also Arrington v. Wong*, 237 F.3d 1066, 1072 (9th Cir. 2001) (reasoning through negative implication that a hospital may not divert an ambulance if it is *not* in diversionary status).

[15] *Morales v. Sociedad Española de Auxilio Mutuo y Beneficencia*, 524 F.3d 54 (1st Cir. 2008) (cert. denied *Sociedad Espanola v. Morales*, 77 U.S.LW. 3396 (2009)).

[16] *Id.* at 59-62.

[17] 42 C.F.R. § 489.24(b). Prior to the promulgation of these regulations, the Seventh Circuit had held that contacting a hospital via telemetry alone does not invoke EMTALA. *Johnson v. Univ. of Chicago Hosps.*, 982 F.2d 230 (7th Cir. 1993). These regulations are consonant with that holding.

[18] *Phillips v. Hillcrest Med. Ctr.*, 244 F.3d 790 (10th Cir. 2001) (noting that EMTALA was not enacted to create a federal medical malpractice standard).

[19] 42 U.S.C. § 1395dd(a). Screening exams may vary based upon a hospital's capabilities and the nature of an individual's request. 42 C.F.R. § 489.24(a)(i) and (c).

[20] *Correa v. Hosp. San Francisco*, 69 F.3d 1184 (1st Cir. 1995), *Baber v. Hosp. Corp. of America*, 977 F.2d 872 (4th Cir. 1992), *Marshall v. E. Carroll Parish Hosp. Serv.*, 134 F.3d 319 (5th Cir. 1998), *Summers v. Baptist Med. Ctr. Arkadelphia*, 91 F.3d 1132 (8th Cir. 1996), *Jackson v. E. Bay Hosp.*, 246 F.3d 1248 (9th Cir. 2001), *Holcomb v. Monahan*, 30 F.3d 116 (1 1th Cir. 1994), *Gatewood v. Wash. Healthcare Corp.*, 933 F.2d 1037 (D. C. Cir. 1991).

[21] *Cleland v. Bronson Health Care Group, Inc.*, 917 F2d 266, 272 (6th Cir. 1990). Gender, race, nationality, financial insolvency, bias against a particular medical condition, and personal animosity were examples of improper motivation offered by the *Cleland* court.

[22] 42 C.F.R. § 489.24(f). Examples of specialized equipment or expertise include burn units, shock-trauma units, neonatal intensive care units, or regional referral centers.

[23] 42 U.S.C. § 1395dd(b)(1) and 42 C.F.R. § 489.24(a)(1)(ii).

[24] *Bryant v. Adventist*, *infra* note 28 at 1166.

[25] 42 C.F.R. § 489.24(b).

[26] 42 U.S.C. § 1395dd(b)(1)(A).

[27] *Roberts v. Galen*, 525 U.S. 249, 252-3 (1999). The Court expressly declined to decide whether the "improper motive" requirement was required with respect to EMTALA's screening provisions. *Id.* at 253 n. 1. *See also supra* notes 20-2 1 and accompanying text.

[28] *Bryan v. Rectors & Visitors of the Univ. of Virginia*, 95 F.3d 349, 352 (4th Cir. 1996), *Bryant v. Adventist Health Sys.*, 289 F.3d 1162, 1168-1169 (9th Cir. 2002), *Harry v. Marchant*, 291 F.3d 767 (11th Cir. 2002).

[29] *Thornton v. Southwest Detroit Hosp.*, 895 F.2d 1131, 1135 (6th Cir. 1990).

[30] The Sixth Circuit argued in dictum that if EMTALA did not apply to inpatients, hospitals could avoid EMTALA liability by admitting, and immediately discharging, a patient. *Id.* at 1135.

[31] *Roberts v. Galen*, 525 U.S. at 253-4 n.2.

[32] Transcript of Oral Argument at 17-20, *Roberts v. Galen, supra* note 27. The Solicitor General also argued that the question of inpatient status had not been properly raised in the courts below.

[33] Notice of Proposed Rule, 67 Fed. Reg. 31,403, 31,475-6 (May 9, 2002).

[34] *Bryant v. Adventist Health Sys.*, 289 F.3d at 1168-1169.

[35] Notice of Final Rule, 68 Fed. Reg. 53,221, 53,243-5 (Sept. 9, 2003). Comments also expressed concerns that EMTALA would usurp existing protections for inpatients.

[36] 42 C.F.R. § 489.24(d)(2). Inpatients are still protected by other Medicare conditions of participation. Persons admitted for elective treatment or diagnosis are still covered under EMTALA. *Id.*

[37] 73 Fed. Reg. 48,656-61.

[38] *See supra* note 22 and accompanying text.

[39] 42 C.F.R. 489.24(f)(2).

[40] *Moses v. Providence Hosp. & Med. Ctrs., Inc.*, 561 F.3d 573, 582 (6th Cir. 2009). The defendant in this case has sought review by the Supreme Court.

[41] *Id.* at 583.

[42] *Id.*

[43] *In re Baby K*, 16 F.3d 590 (4th Cir. 1994).

[44] *Id.* at 596-7.

[45] *Id.* EMTALA explicitly preempts any state laws that directly conflict with EMTALA's provisions. 42 U.S.C. § 1395dd(f). The Fourth Circuit later clarified *Baby K's* holding in *Bryan v. Univ. of Virginia*, ruling that EMTALA only mandates treating a patient's emergency medical condition, not the patient's general medical condition. *Bryan v. Univ. of Virginia*, 95 F.3d at 352. Therefore, had the hospital admitted Baby K after stabilizing her emergency respiratory distress, it would not have been required to then treat her underlying anencephaly beyond warmth and nutrition. *Id.*

[46] 42 C.F.R. § 489.24(e)(2).

[47] 42 C.F.R. § 489.24(e)(1)(ii)(B).

[48] *Moses v. Providence Hosp. & Med. Ctrs., Inc.*, 561 F.3d at 579-582.

[49] H.Rept. 99-24 1, at 6.

[50] *Moses*, 2009 U.S. App. LEXIS 7049, at 17-19.

[51] 42 U.S.C. § 1395dd(d)(2)(A) (emphasis added).

In: Issues in Providing Emergency Medical Care ISBN: 978-1-61761-595-5
Editor: Mary E. Mathers

Chapter 2

HOSPITAL EMERGENCY DEPARTMENTS: CROWDING CONTINUES TO OCCUR, AND SOME PATIENTS WAIT LONGER THAN RECOMMENDED TIME FRAMES

United States Government Accountability Office

WHY GAO DID THIS STUDY

Hospital emergency departments are a major part of the nation's health care safety net. Of the estimated 119 million visits to U.S. emergency departments in 2006, over 40 percent were paid for by federally-supported programs. These programs—Medicare, Medicaid, and the State Children's Health Insurance Program—are administered by the Department of Health and Human Services (HHS). There have been reports of crowded conditions in emergency departments, often associated with adverse effects on patient quality of care. In 2003, GAO reported that most emergency departments in metropolitan areas experienced some degree of crowding (*Hospital Emergency Departments: Crowded Conditions Vary among Hospitals and Communities*, GAO-03-460). For example, two out of every three metropolitan hospitals reported going on ambulance diversion—asking ambulances to bypass their emergency departments and instead transport patients to other facilities.

GAO was asked to examine information made available since 2003 on emergency department crowding. GAO examined three indicators of emergency department crowding—ambulance diversion, wait times, and patient boarding—and factors that contribute to crowding. To conduct this work, GAO reviewed national data; conducted a literature review of 197 articles; and interviewed officials from HHS and professional and research organizations, and individual subject-matter experts.

What GAO Found

Emergency department crowding continues to occur in hospital emergency departments according to national data, articles we reviewed, and officials we interviewed. National data show that hospitals continue to divert ambulances, with about one-fourth of hospitals reporting going on diversion at least once in 2006. National data also indicate that wait times in the emergency department increased, and in some cases exceeded recommended time frames. For example, the average wait time to see a physician for emergent patients—those patients who should be seen in 1 to 14 minutes—was 37 minutes in 2006, more than twice as long as recommended for their level of urgency. Boarding of patients in the emergency department who are awaiting transfer to an inpatient bed or another facility continues to be reported as a problem in articles we reviewed and by officials we interviewed, but national data on the extent to which this occurs are limited. Moreover, some of the articles we reviewed discussed strategies to address crowding, but these strategies have not been assessed on a state or national level.

Articles we reviewed and individual subject-matter experts we interviewed reported that a lack of access to inpatient beds continues to be the main factor contributing to emergency department crowding, although additional factors may contribute. One reason for a lack of access to inpatient beds is competition between hospital admissions from the emergency department and scheduled admissions—for example, for elective surgeries, which may be more profitable for the hospital. Additional factors may contribute to emergency department crowding, including patients' lack of access to primary care services or a shortage of available on-call specialists.

In commenting on a draft of this chapter, HHS noted that the report demonstrates that emergency department wait times are continuing to increase and frequently exceed national standards. HHS also provided technical comments, which we incorporated as appropriate.

Average Wait Time to See a Physician and Percentage of Visits in Which Wait Time to See a Physician Exceeded Recommended Time Frames by Acuity Level, 2006

Patient acuity level[a] (recommended time frame)	Average wait time in minutes	Percentage of visits in which wait time exceeded recommended time frames
Immediate (less than 1 minute)	28	73.9
Emergent (1 to 14 minutes)	37	50.4
Urgent (15 to 60 minutes)	50	20.7
Semiurgent (greater than 1 to 2 hours)	68	13.3
Nonurgent (greater than 2 to 24 hours)	76	—[b]

Source: GAO analysis of data from HHS's National Center for Health Statistics (NCHS).

Notes: Information on the standard error associated with estimates of averages is found in the report

[a]Acuity levels describe the recommended time a patient should wait to be seen by a physician. NCHS developed acuity levels based on a five-level emergency severity index recommended by the Emergency Nurses Association.

[b]In 2006, no emergency departments reported visits with wait times in excess of 24 hours.

ABBREVIATIONS

ACEP	American College of Emergency Physicians
AHRQ	Agency for Healthcare Research and Quality
DRG	diagnosis-related group
HHS	Department of Health and Human Services
IOM	Institute of Medicine
NCHS	National Center for Health Statistics
NHAMCS	National Hospital Ambulatory Medical Care Survey

April 30, 2009

The Honorable Max Baucus
Chairman
Committee on Finance
United States Senate

Dear Mr. Chairman:

Open 24 hours a day, 7 days a week, hospital emergency departments are a major part of the nation's health care safety net. Of the estimated 119 million visits to U.S. emergency departments in 2006, over 40 percent were paid for by federally-supported programs.[1] These programs— Medicare, Medicaid, and the State Children's Health Insurance Program[2]— are administered by the Department of Health and Human Services (HHS). Emergency department staff report being under increasing pressure, and concerns have been raised that they face challenges in providing timely and effective emergency medical care. For example, considerable attention has been given to reports of ambulance diversion—that is, emergency departments requesting that ambulances that would normally bring patients to their hospitals go instead to other hospitals that are presumably less crowded. Concerns have also been raised about the frequency of patients remaining in the emergency department—taking up staff and resources—after the decision has been made to admit them to the hospital or transfer them to another facility, a practice known as boarding. In addition, reports of long wait times in emergency departments have led to concerns of potential adverse effects on the quality of care for patients, such as prolonged pain and suffering.

We have reported on the extent of crowding in emergency departments and factors contributing to crowding. In 2003, we reported results from our survey of more than 2,000 hospitals with emergency departments located in metropolitan areas of the country and from our site visits to communities where media and other sources had reported problems with emergency department crowding.[3] Using three indicators of crowding— diversion, patients leaving the emergency department before a medical evaluation (presumably due to long wait times in the emergency department), and boarding—we found that while most emergency departments across the country experienced some degree of crowding,[4] crowding was much more pronounced in some hospitals and areas than in others. Generally, hospitals that reported the most problems with emergency department crowding were in metropolitan areas with populations of 2.5 million or more. We also found that crowding is a complex issue and that one key factor contributing to crowding at many hospitals was the inability of hospitals to move admitted patients out of emergency departments and into inpatient beds. Reasons given for why hospitals did not have the capacity to meet demand for inpatient beds from emergency department patients included financial pressures leading to limited hospital capacity and competition between admissions from the emergency department and scheduled admissions, such as for elective surgery. Finally, we reported on strategies that were implemented to address emergency department crowding in the six communities that we visited; however, we found that studies assessing the effect of these efforts were limited.

Since our 2003 report, Congress and others have raised concerns that hospital emergency departments are continuing to experience crowded conditions that could potentially compromise the nation's ability to provide effective emergency medical care. For example, in September 2003 the Institute of Medicine (IOM) convened a committee to examine, among other things, emergency department crowding.[5] In addition, in June 2007 the House Committee on Oversight and Government Reform held a hearing at which experts in hospital emergency care testified on the state of the nation's emergency care. Given this continued interest, you asked to us to report on information made available with respect to emergency department crowding since we issued our 2003 report. Specifically, this chapter examines information made available about (1) three indicators of emergency department crowding—ambulance diversion, wait times,[6] and patient boarding, and (2) factors that contribute to emergency department crowding.

To conduct this work, we reviewed national data, conducted a literature review, and interviewed federal and other officials. First, we obtained and reviewed national data on emergency department diversion and wait times for 2001 through 2006 from the National Center for Health Statistics (NCHS)[7] and data on hospital admissions—which were related to factors of crowding—from the Agency for Healthcare Research and Quality (AHRQ).[8] We obtained nationally-representative data from NCHS and AHRQ beginning with 2001 because these data became publicly available in 2003 or later, meeting the criterion for inclusion in our analysis. At the time we conducted our analysis, the most recent year for which data were available from NCHS and AHRQ was 2006. In addition, some data from NCHS were not available for all years between 2001 and 2006 because of revisions made by NCHS to questions on surveys used to collect information or a low response rate to certain questions on these surveys. As part of our review of available national data on emergency department diversion and wait times, we analyzed wait times in the emergency department using NCHS's data on recommended time for a patient to see a physician based on patient acuity levels.[9] We also reviewed national data on emergency department utilization to set up a context for our work. In this chapter, we present NCHS estimates; for those cases in which we report an increase or other comparison of these estimates, NCHS tested the differences and found them statistically significant.[10] To assess the reliability of national data from NCHS and AHRQ, we discussed the data with agency officials and reviewed the methods they used for collecting and reporting these data. We resolved discrepancies we found between the data provided to us and data in published reports by corresponding with officials from NCHS to obtain sufficient explanations for the differences. Based on these steps, we determined that these data were sufficiently reliable for our purposes.

We also conducted a literature review of 197 articles, including articles published in peer-reviewed and other periodicals, publications from professional and research organizations, and reports issued by federal and state agencies. In examining the information made available since 2003 about indicators of crowding during our literature review, we analyzed articles for what was reported on the effect of crowding on patient quality of care and on proposed strategies to address crowding. We reviewed 197 articles, publications, and reports (which we call articles)[11] on emergency department crowding published on or between January 1, 2003, and August 31, 2008. These included articles reporting on results of surveys conducted by the American College of Emergency Physicians (ACEP) and the American Hospital Association that provided information on ambulance diversion that was not available from NCHS. A complete bibliography for the literature review can be viewed at GAO-09-348SP.

Finally, we interviewed officials from federal agencies and one state agency, professional and research organizations, other hospital-related organizations, and individual subject-matter experts to obtain and review information on indicators of emergency department crowding and factors that contribute to crowding. We interviewed federal officials from HHS's Centers for Medicare & Medicaid Services and the Office of the Assistant Secretary for Preparedness and Response, and officials from NCHS and AHRQ who have conducted research on emergency department utilization and crowding. We also interviewed officials from professional and research organizations, including ACEP, the American Hospital Association, the American Medical Association, the Center for Studying Health System Change, and the Society for Academic Emergency Medicine. Some of the officials from ACEP and the Society for Academic Emergency Medicine whom we interviewed have also published research in peer-reviewed journals. Additionally, we interviewed hospital-related organizations, including those involved in hospital accreditation and in developing quality measures for hospital emergency department care, and officials from the Massachusetts Department of Public Health. Finally, we interviewed three individual subject-matter experts knowledgeable about emergency department crowding. Additional information about our methodology can be found in appendix I.

We conducted this performance audit from May 2008 through April 2009 in accordance with generally accepted government auditing standards. Those standards require that we plan and perform the audit to obtain sufficient, appropriate evidence to provide a reasonable basis for our findings and conclusions based on our audit objectives. We believe that the evidence obtained provides a reasonable basis for our findings and conclusions based on our audit objectives.

BACKGROUND

Thousands of emergency departments operate in the United States, seeing millions of patients each year. In our 2003 report on emergency department crowding, we reported on the extent of crowding in metropolitan areas. Researchers have used three indicators—diversion, wait times, and boarding—in examining emergency department crowding.

Emergency Department Utilization

Between 2001 and 2006, according to NCHS estimates, the number of emergency departments operating in the United States ranged from about 4,600 to about 4,900.[12] During the same period, the estimated number of visits to U.S. emergency departments exceeded 107 million visits each year, ranging from about 107 million visits in 2001 to about 119 million visits in 2006. (See table 1.)

Most hospitals with emergency departments are located in metropolitan areas, and the majority of emergency department visits occurred in metropolitan areas of the United States.[13] In 2006, about two-thirds of hospitals with emergency departments were located in metropolitan areas compared to about one-third in nonmetropolitan areas. In the same year, about 101 million (85 percent) of the approximately 119 million emergency department visits occurred in metropolitan areas compared to about 18 million (15 percent) visits in nonmetropolitan areas. (See figure1.)

Patients come to the emergency department with illnesses or injuries of varying severity, referred to as acuity level. Each acuity level corresponds to a recommended time frame for being seen by a physician—for example, patients with immediate conditions should be seen within 1 minute and patients with emergent conditions should be seen within 1 to 14 minutes. In 2006, urgent patients—patients who are recommended to be seen by a physician within 15 to 60 minutes—accounted for the highest percentage of visits to the emergency department. (See figure 2.)

Table 1. Number of Emergency Departments and Emergency Department Visits in 2001 Through 2006

In thousands						
	2001	**2002**	**2003**	**2004**	**2005**	**2006**
Total number of emergency departments operating	4.6	4.9	4.7	4.7	4.6	4.8
Total annual emergency department visit volume	107,490	110,155	113,903	110,216	115,323	119,191

Source: GAO analysis of NCHS data.

Note: All estimates in this table are nationally representative. NCHS estimates the number of hospitals with an emergency department in the United States that is staffed and operated 24 hours a day.

The expected sources of payment[14] reported for patients receiving emergency department services also vary. For example, from 2001 through 2006 patients with private insurance accounted for the highest number and percentage of visits to the emergency department. During the same period, the percentage of uninsured patients[15] seeking care in emergency departments ranged between 15 and 17 percent of total visits, and the percentage of patients visiting emergency departments with Medicare ranged between 14 and 16 percent. See appendix II for additional data on expected sources of payment and emergency department utilization.

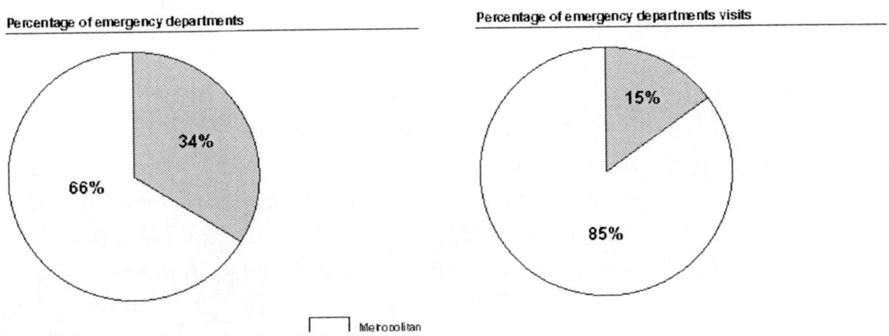

Source: GAO analysis of NCHS data.

Figure 1. Percentage of Emergency Departments and Emergency Department Visits in Metropolitan and Nonmetropolitan Areas in 2006

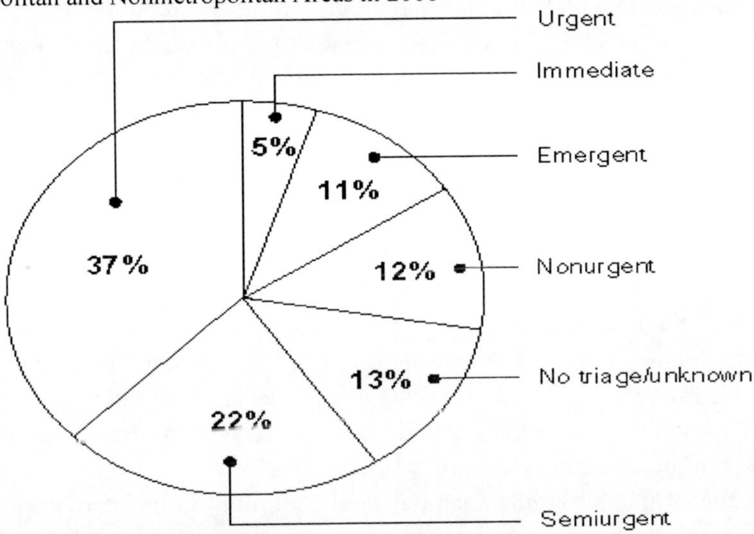

Source: GAO analysis of NCHS data.

Note: NCHS developed time-based acuity levels based on a five-level emergency severity index recommended by the Emergency Nurses Association. The acuity levels describe the recommended amount of time a patient should wait to be seen by a physician. The recommended time frames to see a physician are less than 1 minute for immediate patients, between 1 and 14 minutes for emergent patients, between 15 minutes and 1 hour for urgent patients, greater than 1 hour to 2 hours for semiurgent patients, and greater than 2 hours to 24 hours for nonurgent patients.

Figure 2. Percentage of Emergency Department Visits by Acuity Level in 2006

Key Findings from the 2003 GAO Report on Emergency Department Crowding

In 2003, using three indicators that point to situations in which crowding is likely occurring—diversion,[16] patients leaving before a medical evaluation, and boarding—we reported that emergency department crowding varied nationwide. We also reported that crowding was more pronounced in certain types of communities, and that crowding occurred more frequently in hospitals located in metropolitan areas with larger populations, higher population growth, and higher levels of uninsurance. We reported that crowding was more evident in certain types of hospitals, such as in hospitals with higher numbers of staffed beds, teaching hospitals, public hospitals, and hospitals designated as certified trauma centers.

In terms of factors that contribute to crowding, we reported that crowding is a complex issue and no single factor tends to explain why crowding occurs. However, we found that one key factor contributing to crowding was the availability of inpatient beds for patients admitted to the hospital from the emergency department. Reasons given by hospital officials and researchers we interviewed for not always having enough inpatient beds to meet demand from emergency patients included economic factors that influence hospitals' capability to meet periodic spikes in demand and emergency department admissions competing with other admissions for inpatient beds. Other additional factors cited by researchers and hospital officials as contributing to crowding included the lack of availability of physicians and other community services—such as psychiatric services— and the fact that emergency patients are older, have more complex conditions, and have more treatment and tests provided in the emergency department than in prior years.

Further, we reported that hospitals and communities had conducted a wide range of activities to manage crowding in emergency departments, but that problems with crowding persisted in spite of these efforts. These activities included efforts to expand capacity and increase efficiency in hospitals, and community activities to implement systems and rules to manage diversion. These efforts were unable to reverse crowding trends at hospital emergency departments, and we found that studies assessing the effect of these efforts were limited.

Indicators of Emergency Department Crowding

Researchers use the indicators we reported on in 2003 to point to situations in which crowding is likely occurring in emergency departments.[17] These indicators can point to when crowding is likely occurring but they also have limitations. For example, patients boarding in the emergency department can indicate that the department's capacity to treat additional patients is diminished, but it is possible for several patients to be boarding while the emergency department has available treatment spaces to see additional patients. Table 2 provides the definition of the three indicators of emergency department crowding we reviewed in this chapter—diversion, wait times, and boarding—and lists the usefulness and limitations of using these indicators to gauge crowding. Regarding wait times, in our 2003 report, we used "left before a medical evaluation" as an indicator of crowding related to long wait times in an emergency department. Since we issued our report in 2003, researchers have used intervals of wait times—including the length of time to see a physician and the total length of time a patient is in the emergency department—to indicate when an emergency department is crowded. As a result, for this chapter, we examined wait times more broadly, including data on the time for patients to see a physician, length of stay in the emergency department, and visits in which the patient left before a medical evaluation.[18]

Researchers have developed a conceptual model to analyze the factors that contribute to emergency department crowding and develop potential solutions.[19] This model partitions emergency department crowding into three interdependent components: input, throughput, and output. Although factors in many different parts of the health care system may contribute to emergency department crowding, the model focuses on crowding from the perspective of the emergency department. (See figure 3.)

Researchers have used the input-throughput-output model to explain the connection between factors that contribute to emergency department crowding and indicators of crowding. The three indicators of emergency department crowding—diversion, wait times, and boarding—are most directly related to the input, throughput, and output components, respectively, of the model; but the causes of these indicators can relate to other components. For example, a hospital emergency department might experience long wait times—an indicator associated with the throughput component—because of delays in patients receiving laboratory results (related to throughput) or because staff are busy caring for patients boarding in the emergency department due to a lack of access to inpatient beds (related to output). Similarly, an emergency department may divert ambulances (related to input) because the emergency department is full due to the inability of hospital staff to move admitted patients to hospital inpatient beds (related to output).

Table 2. Indicators of Emergency Department Crowding

Indicator	Definition	Usefulness	Limitations
Ambulanc e diversion	Hospitals request that ambulances bypass their emergency departments and transport patients to other medical facilities.	For emergency depart-ments where local rules permit diversion, diver-sion is an indicator of how often emergency departments believe that they cannot safely handle additional ambulance patients.	The number of hours on diversion is a potentially imprecise measure of crowding because whether a hospital can go on diversion and the circu-mstances under which it can do so vary from location to location, according to both individual hospital policy and com-munitywide guidelines or rules.
Wait times	Intervals of wait time include the amount of time a patient waits in the emergency depart-ment to see a physic-cian, the percentage of visits in which patients left before a medical evaluation, and the total length of time a patient spends in the emergency department.	Long wait times can occur when an emergency department is crowded and unable to treat patients waiting to be seen in a reasonable amount of time. Excessive wait time is the most common reason patients leave the emergency department before being treated.	Since emergency depart-ment staff triage patie-nts, those with condit-ions that do not present an immediate emergency generally wait the lon-gest. These patients may also be most likely to tire of waiting and leave before receiving a medi-cal evaluation. In addit-ion, because there are several ways to measure wait times, it can be difficult to compare wait times across hospitals or studies.
Patient boarding	A patient remains in the emergency depart-ment after the decis-ion to admit or transfer the patient has been made, for example because an inpatient bed elsewhere in the hospital is not yet available.	Patients boarding in the emergency department take up space and reso-urces that could be used to treat other emergency department patients. Boarding is an indicator that an emergency department's capacity to treat additional patients is diminished.	Boarding does not alwa-ys indicate that an emer-gency department is cro-wded since it is possible for an emergency depart-ment to be boarding pat-ients while also having available treatment spaces.

Source: GAO.

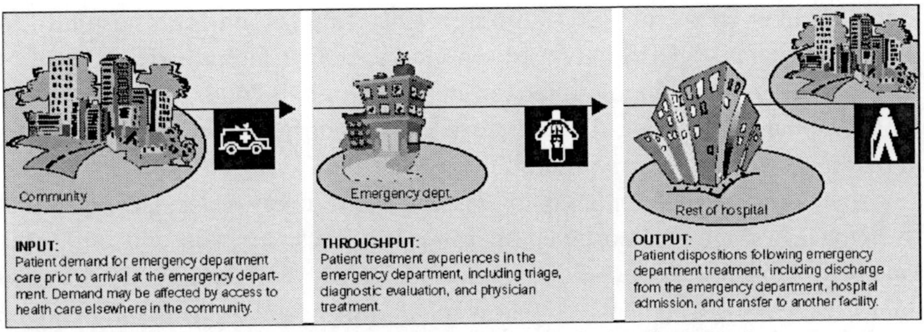

Source: GAO analysis of published literature, Art Explosion (graphics).

Figure 3. Input-Throughput-Output Model of Emergency Department Crowding

According to Indicators, Emergency Department Crowding Continues

We found that ambulance diversions continue, wait times have increased, and reports of boarding in hospital emergency departments persist. Articles we reviewed also reported on the effect of crowding on quality of care and on strategies proposed to address crowding.

Hospitals Continue to Divert Ambulances

National data show that the diversion of ambulances continues to occur, but that the percentage of hospitals that go on diversion and the average number of hours hospitals spend on diversion varied by year. According to NCHS estimates, in 2003, 45 percent of U.S. hospitals reported going on diversion, and in 2004 through 2006, between 25 and 27 percent reported doing so. Of hospitals that reported going on diversion, the average number of hours they reported spending on diversion varied with an average of 276 hours in 2003 and an average of 473 hours in 2006.[20] (See table 3.) NCHS officials provided the percentage of missing diversion data for each year, which ranged from 3.75 percent in 2003 to 29.1 percent in 2005.[21] NCHS officials, however, were unable to provide an explanation for the variation of the percentage of hospitals going on diversion in the United States and average hours U.S. hospitals reported spending on diversion for these years. NCHS reported that hospitals in metropolitan areas spent more time on diversion than hospitals in nonmetroplitan areas in 2003 through 2004: almost half of hospitals in metropolitan areas NCHS surveyed reported spending more than 1 percent of their total operating time on diversion in 2003 through 2004,[22] compared to 1 in 10 hospitals in nonmetropolitan areas.[23] Some hospitals, however, reported that their state or local laws prohibit diversion.[24]

Other articles that reported on results from surveys also indicated that diversion has continued to occur in some hospitals. In 2006 and 2007, the American Hospital Association conducted surveys of community hospital chief executive officers that asked how much time hospitals spent on diversion in the previous year.[25] The results from these surveys show that some hospitals reported going on diversion.[26] In both American Hospital Association surveys, urban hospitals more often reported diversion hours than rural hospitals. For example, among hospitals responding to the 2006 American Hospital Association survey, about 64 percent of respondents from urban hospitals reported going on diversion, compared to about 17 percent of respondents from rural hospitals. In addition, articles reporting on emergency department crowding in California[27] and Maryland[28] also found that diversion continues to occur and that the time hospitals spent on diversion varied.[29]

Wait Times Have Increased and in Some Cases Exceeded Recommended Time Frames

National data from NCHS indicate that wait times in the emergency department have increased and in some cases exceeded recommended time frames. For example, the average wait time to see a physician increased from 46 minutes in 2003 to 56 minutes in 2006.[30] Average wait times also increased for patients in some acuity levels.[31] (See figure 4.) For emergent patients,[32] the average wait time to see a physician increased from 23 minutes to 37 minutes, more than twice as long as recommended for their level of acuity. For immediate, emergent, urgent, and semiurgent patients, NCHS estimates show that some patients were not seen within the recommended time frames for their acuity level.

Table 3. Percentage of Hospitals That Reported Going on Diversion, and Average Hours Hospitals Spent on Diversion in 2003 through 2006

	2003	2004	2005	2006
Percentage of hospitals that reported going on diversion[a]	44.5	24.8	26.1	27.3
Average hours spent on diversion[b]	276	516	323	473

Source: GAO analysis of NCHS data.

Notes: All estimates in this table are nationally representative.

[a] Diversion data were missing for 3.75 percent of emergency departments in 2003, for 24.1 percent in 2004, for 29.1 percent in 2005, and for 20.5 percent in 2006.

[b] Average is the estimated mean. Standard error is a statistic used to calculate the range of values that express the possible difference between the sample estimate and the actual population value. The standard error for average hours spent on diversion was 42 for 2003, 70 for 2004, 58 for 2005, and 73 for 2006.

Acuity level[a] (recommended time frame)	Average wait time in mintues[b]		Percentage of visits in which wait time exceeded recommended time frames[c]	
	2003	2006	2003	2006
Immediate[d] (less than 1 minute)	23	28	37.5	73.9
Emergent[d,e] (1 to 14 minutes)		37		50.4
Urgent[e] (15 to 60 minutes)	42	50	17.0	20.7
Semiurgent[e] (greater than 1 hour to 2 hours)	60	68	9.6	13.3
Nonurgent (greater than 2 hours to 24 hours)	69	76	–[f]	–[f]
No triage[g,h]	48	45	–[i]	–[i]
Unknown[h]		66		–[i]
All acuity levels	46	56	–[i]	–[i]

Source: GAO analysis of NCHS data.

Notes: All estimates in this figure are nationally representative.

Figure 4. Average Wait Time to See a Physician, and Percentage of Visits in Which Wait Time to See a Physician Exceeded Recommended Time Frames by Acuity Level in 2003 and 2006

[a] NCHS developed time-based acuity levels based on a five-level emergency severity index recommended by the Emergency Nurses Association. The acuity levels describe the recommended amount of time a patient should wait to be seen by a physician.

[b] Average is the estimated mean. Standard error is a statistic used to calculate the range of values that express the possible difference between the sample estimate and the

actual population value. The standard error for average wait time to see a physician in 2003 ranged from 2 to 5 minutes. The standard error for average wait time to see a physician in 2006 ranged from 2 to 6 minutes with the exception of a standard error of 11 minutes for unknown acuity level.

[c] The numbers in these columns represent the percentage of visits with wait times exceeding the recommended amount of time for their acuity level.

[d] NCHS added an immediate wait time category to the NHAMCS survey instrument starting in 2005. For 2003, the emergent category was defined as a visit with a recommended wait time of less than 15 minutes.

[e] According to NCHS, from 2003 to 2006 the increase in average wait time to see a physician for visits by emergent, urgent, and semiurgent patients was statistically significant.

[f] For 2003, wait times in excess of 24 hours were not able to be reported on the NHAMCS survey instrument. For 2006, no emergency departments in the sample reported visits with wait times in excess of 24 hours. As a result, the percentages of nonurgent visits with wait times exceeding the recommended time frame were not available.

[g] A visit in which there is no mention of an acuity rating or triage level in the medical record, the hospital did not perform triage, or the patient was dead on arrival.

[h] For 2003, the NHAMCS survey instrument grouped no triage and unknown acuity level into a single category.

[I] Visits with no triage reported or an unknown acuity level did not have an associated recommended amount of time to see a physician. Therefore, percentages of visits with wait times exceeding recommended time frames could not be calculated for these categories of visits, or all acuity levels combined.

The average wait time to see a physician increased in emergency departments in metropolitan areas, and wait times were longer in emergency departments in metropolitan areas than in nonmetropolitan areas in 2006. In metropolitan-area emergency departments, the average wait time to see a physician increased from 51 minutes in 2003 to 60 minutes in 2006. In nonmetropolitan-area emergency departments, the average wait time to see a physician was estimated to be about 26 minutes in 2003 and 33 minutes in 2006.[33] According to NCHS data, the average length of stay in the emergency department and the percentage of visits in which patients left before a medical evaluation also increased. (See table 4.) See appendix IV for additional information about wait times in the emergency department.

Table 4. Average Length of Stay in the Emergency Department, in Minutes, and Percentage of Visits in Which Patients Left before a Medical Evaluation in 2001 and 2006

	2001[a]	2006[b]
Average length of stay in the emergency department, in minutes		
All hospitals	178	199
Hospitals in metropolitan areas[c]	189	211
Hospitals in nonmetropolitan areas[c]	131	139
Percentage of visits in which patients left before a medical evaluation[d]		
All hospitals	1.5	2.0
Hospitals in metropolitan areas[c]	1.7	2.2
Hospitals in nonmetropolitan areas[c]	0.6	0.9

Source: GAO analysis of NCHS data.

Notes: All estimates in this table are nationally representative.

[a] Standard error is a statistic used to calculate the range of values that express the possible difference between the sample estimate and the actual population value. The standard error for the average length of stay in the emergency department in 2001 ranged from 4 to 5 minutes.

[b] The standard error for the average length of stay in the emergency department in 2006 ranged from 5 to 7 minutes.

[c] *Metropolitan* describes hospitals identified by NCHS as located in a metropolitan statistical area and *nonmetropolitan* describes hospitals identified by NCHS as not located in a metropolitan statistical area.

[d] NCHS defines the percentage of visits in which patients left before a medical evaluation as the percentage of visits in which the patient left after triage but before receiving any medical care.

Boarding Continues to Be Reported, but National Data on Boarding Have Been Limited

More than 25 percent of the 197 articles we reviewed discuss the practice of boarding patients in emergency departments, and officials we interviewed noted that the practice of boarding continues. For example, in 2006 IOM reported that boarding continues to occur and has become a typical practice in hospitals nationwide, with the most boarding occurring at large urban hospitals.[34] One article published in a peer-reviewed journal reported that it is not unusual for critically ill patients to board in the emergency department.[35] In addition, officials we interviewed noted that the practice of boarding patients in emergency departments persists. In particular, officials from the Center for Studying Health System Change noted that boarding still occurs in emergency departments and continues to be one of the main indicators of emergency department crowding. Officials from ACEP noted that boarding continues to occur in emergency departments nationwide and remains a concern for emergency physicians and their patients.

National data on the boarding of patients in the emergency department, however, have been limited. In 2006, IOM reported that hospital data systems do not adequately monitor or measure patient flow, and therefore may be limited in their ability to capture data on boarding. For example, few systems distinguish between when a patient is ready to move to another location for care and when that move actually takes place.[36] In addition, from 2001 to 2006, NCHS did not collect data on boarding because, according to NCHS officials, data on boarding were not easily obtained from patient records. A question about emergency department boarding was added to NCHS's NHAMCS questionnaire in 2007; however, data from this survey were not available at the time we conducted our analysis. Other articles that reported on results of surveys conducted by professional associations supported officials' statements that boarding has been widespread. For example, in an article reporting on a 2005 ACEP survey of emergency department directors with a 30 percent response rate, 996 of the 1,328 respondents reported that they boarded patients for at least 4 hours on a daily basis and more than 200 respondents reported that they did so for more than 10 patients per day on average.[37]

Articles and Officials Discussed the Effect of Crowding and Strategies for Decreasing Diversion, Wait Times, and BoardingArticles and Officials Discussed the Effect of Crowding and Strategies for Decreasing Diversion, Wait Times, and Boarding

Ten of the articles we reviewed and officials from ACEP and the Society for Academic Emergency Medicine whom we interviewed raised concerns about the adverse effect of diversion, wait times, or boarding on the quality of patient care, but quantitative evidence of this effect has been limited. Officials from ACEP reported that research has begun to analyze the effect of crowding on patient quality of care, and that anecdotal reports indicate patients are being harmed. Ten of the articles we reviewed discussed the effect of diversion, wait times, or boarding on quality of care. One of these articles, the 2006 IOM report, noted that ambulance diversion could lead to catastrophic delays in treatment for seriously ill or injured patients and that boarding may enhance the potential for errors, delays in treatment, and diminished quality of care.[38] Other articles—some of which were published in peer-reviewed journals—also discussed the effect of crowding on the quality of patient care, including the following:

- An examination of the relationship between trauma death rates and hospital diversion, which suggested that death rates for trauma patients at two hospitals may be correlated with diversion at these hospitals.[39]
- A review of 24 hospital emergency departments that suggested when an emergency department experienced an increase in the number of patients leaving before a medical evaluation, fewer patients with pneumonia at the emergency department received antibiotics within the recommended 4 hours.[40]
- Information from a database of 90 hospitals that showed patients who were boarded in the emergency department for more than 6 hours before being transferred to the hospital's intensive care unit had an almost 5 percent higher in-hospital mortality rate than those who were boarded for less than 6 hours.[41]
- Five other articles reported potential associations between diversion, boarding, and wait times and decreased quality of patient care, including articles on the effect of increasing wait times for nonurgent patients in the emergency department and delayed treatment time for those patients who left before a medical evaluation.

While these studies support the widely held assertion that emergency department crowding adversely affects the quality of patient care, a 2006 National Health Policy Forum[42] report stated that the consequences of crowded emergency departments on quality of care have not been studied comprehensively and therefore little quantitative evidence is available to confirm this assumption.[43] Officials from the Society for Academic Emergency Medicine reported that diversion, wait times, and boarding can contribute to reduced quality of care and worse patient outcomes. In addition, officials from both ACEP and the Society for Academic Emergency Medicine noted that additional studies about the effects of diversion, wait times, and boarding on quality of care are needed.

Table 5. Strategies to Address Indicators of Emergency Department Crowding

Strategy	Description of strategy	Assessment of the strategy's effect on indicator(s) of crowding
Strategies related to emergency department input		
Changing dive-rsion policies for the community	A community developed a policy that specified when and under what conditions a hospital was allowed to go on diversion. For example, hospital officials were required to have a process in place that ensured all resources in the hospital were exhausted before going on diversion.	An analysis comparing diversion hours before and after implement-tation of a new diversion policy found that this strategy reduced the hours on diversion by 74 percent in a community of 17 hospitals.[a]
Physician-directed ambul-ance destination-control program	Emergency medical service providers were asked to call a dedicated telephone number that was staffed by attending physici-ans. A destination-control physic-cian determined the optimal pati-ent destination by using patient and system variables as well as emergency medical service providers' and patients' input.	An analysis comparing the diversion hours with and without this program at two hospitals found that this program reduced the hours on diversion by 41 percent at one hospital and 61 percent at the other hospital.[b]
State policy prohibiting diversion	State officials developed a policy that would prohibit hospitals from going on diversion unless the hospital is inoperable under certain conditions.	Officials from the state of Massa-chusetts issued a letter stating that hospitals would no longer be allo-wed to go on diversion unless the hospital was inoperable; however, this policy was implemented in January 2009 and the effect on div-ersion had not yet been analyzed.[c]
Strategies related to emergency department throughput		
A fast-track system	A system that allowed nonurgent patients to be treated in less time	An analysis comparing wait times before and after implementation of

Table 5. (Continued)

Strategy	Description of strategy	Assessment of the strategy's effect on indicator(s) of crowding
	because these patients can be seen by a medical provider other than a physician.	a fast-track system at one hospital found that this strategy reduced both the amount of time patients waited to be seen by a physician and the number of patients who left before a medical evaluation by 50 percent.[d]
A point-of-care testing satellite laboratory	A testing laboratory was set up in close proximity to the emergency department and staffed with a res-earch nurse and laboratory techni-cians. These staff made rounds to the emergency department to coll-ect specimens every 15 minutes and reported results directly to clinicians in the emergency department by telephone or by fax.	An analysis reviewing effects of implementation of a point-of-care testing laboratory in a large univ-ersity-associated urban hospital found that turnaround times for test results were reduced by an average of 87 percent and length of stay in the emergency department decreased for some patients by an average of 41 minutes.[e]
A rapid entry and accelerated care at triage process	A hospital computer system was revised to integrate the emergency department computer system with the computer system for the rest of the hospital, creating a new process when entering data for patients at triage. This process allowed staff to eliminate some of the administer-ative work associated with patients entering the emergency department.	An analysis comparing wait times before and after initiation of this process at one hospital found the process significantly decreased both the rate of patients leaving before being seen and average wait times. The rate of patients leaving before being seen decreased by 3.3 percent and the average wait time decreased by 24 minutes.[f]
Bedside registration	During times when emergency department rooms or beds were available, patients were trans-ported immediately after triage to a patient-care area where they could be simultaneously seen by medical staff and registered at the bedside by a registration clerk.	An analysis of treatment time before and after implementation of bedside registration at one hospital found a small, significant decrease of 13 minutes for treatment time after bedside registration was impl-emented. However, this decrease did not last and treatment time even increased a year after bedside regi-stration was implemented at this hospital.[g]

Table 5. (Continued)

Strategy	Description of strategy	Assessment of the strategy's effect on indicator(s) of crowding
Strategies related to emergency department output		
Increase the capacity of the adult intensive care unit	A hospital expanded the number of beds in its adult intensive care unit from 47 to 67 beds.	An analysis comparing diversion hours before and after the number of adult intensive care unit beds had increased at one hospital found that hours on diversion decreased by 66 percent.[h]
Boarding in the inpatient hallways	A system for moving nonurgent patients admitted to the hospital to inpatient hallways instead of	Not analyzed in published articles[i,j]
	boarding them in emergency department hallways.	
A pull system in the hospital	Staff on inpatient floors played an active role in placing emergency department patients into available beds.	Not analyzed in published articles[j,k]
Streamlining of elective surgery schedules	The strategy will streamline elective surgery schedules to make elective daily admission volume even, and increase the opportunity for emergency department admissions.	Case studies were conducted at se-veral hospitals to determine the inf-luence of reducing the variability of elective surgical scheduling. In one hospital, waiting times for emergent and urgent surgeries has been redu-ced by about 33 percent despite a 30 percent increase in their volumes.[l]

Source: GAO analysis of articles published between January 1, 2003, and August 31, 2008, and interviews.

[a] P. B. Patel et al., "Ambulance Diversion Reduction: the Sacramento Solution," *American Journal of Emergency Medicine*, vol. 24, no. 2 (2006).

[b] M. N. Shah et al., "Description and Evaluation of a Pilot Physician-directed Emergency Medical Services Diversion Control Program," *Academic Emergency Medicine*, vol. 13, no. 1 (2006).

[c] The Commonwealth of Massachusetts, Executive Office of Health and Human Services, Department of Public Health, Circular Letter: DHCQ 08-07-494 (Boston, Mass., July 3, 2008).

[d] M. Sanchez et al ., "Effects of a Fast-Track Area on Emergency Department Performance," *The Journal of Emergency Medicine*, vol. 31, no. 1 (2006).

[e] E. Lee-Lewandrowski et al., "Implementation of a Point-of-Care Satellite Laboratory in the Emergency Department of an Academic Medical Center Impact on Test Turnaround Time and Patient Emergency Department Length of Stay," *Archives of Pathology & Laboratory Medicine*, vol. 127, no. 4 (2003).

[f] T. C. Chan et al., "Impact of Rapid Entry and Accelerated Care at Triage on Reducing Emergency Department Patient Wait Times, Lengths of Stay, and Rate of Left Without Being Seen," *Annals of Emergency Medicine*, vol. 46, no. 6 (2005).

[g] K. M. Takakuwa, F. S. Shofer, and S. B. Abbuhl, "Strategies for Dealing with Emergency Department Overcrowding: A One-Year Study on How Bedside Registration Affects Patient Throughput Times," *The Journal of Emergency Medicine*, vol. 32, no. 4 (2007).

[h] K. J. McConnel et al., "Effect of Increased ICU Capacity on Emergency Department Length of Stay and Ambulance Diversion," *Annals of Emergency Medicine*, vol. 45, no. 5 (2005).

[I] C. Garson et al., "Emergency Department Patient Preferences for Boarding Locations When Hospitals Are at Full Capacity," *Annals of Emergency Medicine*, vol. 51, no. 1 (2008).

[j] While researchers have proposed this strategy to alleviate crowding, analysis has not been published in articles we reviewed to determine if this strategy would decrease boarding.

[k] M. Wilson and K. Nguyen, "Bursting at the Seams, Improving Patient Flow to Help America's Emergency Departments," (Washington, D.C.: Urgent Matters, September 2004), http://www.urgentmatters.org/reports/UM_WhitePaper_BurstingAtTheSeams.pdf (accessed Sept. 30, 2008).

[l] Description of strategy and assessment based on conversation with a subject-matter expert who oversaw these efforts. Additional information is also available on www.bu.edu/mvp (accessed on Apr. 9, 2009).

Articles we reviewed, and officials and an expert we interviewed, discussed a number of strategies that have been proposed, and in some cases tested, that could decrease emergency department crowding. These strategies relate to the three interdependent components—input, throughput, and output—of the model of emergency department crowding developed by researchers. While several of these strategies have been tested, the assessment of their effects has generally been limited to one or a few hospitals and we found no research assessing these strategies on a state or national level. Table 5 outlines some strategies to address emergency department crowding and, to the extent they have been tested, the assessment of their effects on the indicators of crowding.

Available Information Suggests Lack of Access to Inpatient Beds Is the Main Factor Contributing to Crowding, and Other Factors May Also Contribute

Available information suggests that a lack of access to inpatient beds is the main factor contributing to emergency department crowding. Additionally, other factors—a lack of access to primary care, a shortage of available on- call specialists, and difficulties transferring, admitting, or discharging psychiatric patients—have also been reported as contributing to crowding.

Articles and Subject- Matter Experts Have Reported a Lack of Access to Inpatient Beds as the Main Factor Contributing to Crowding

Of the 77 articles we reviewed that discussed factors contributing to crowding, 45 articles reported a lack of access to inpatient beds as a factor contributing to emergency department crowding, with 13 of these articles[44] reporting it was the main factor contributing to crowding.[45] (See table 6.) In addition, two individual subject-matter experts we interviewed also reported a lack of access to inpatient beds as the main factor that contributes to emergency department crowding. When inpatient beds are not available for ill and injured patients who require hospital admission, the emergency department may board them, and these patients take up extra treatment spaces and emergency department resources, leaving fewer resources available for other patients.

One of the reasons that emergency departments are unable to move admitted patients to inpatient beds may be due to competition between emergency department admissions and scheduled hospital admissions— for example, for elective surgical procedures—which we also reported on in 2003. This reason was reported by 9 articles we reviewed and by officials from ACEP, the Society for Academic Emergency Medicine, the Center for Studying Health System Change, and three individual subject- matter experts whom we interviewed. In 2006, IOM reported that hospitals might prefer scheduled admissions over admissions from the emergency department because emergency department admissions are considered to be less profitable.[46] One reason that admissions from the emergency department are considered to be less profitable is because these admissions tend to be for medical conditions, such as heart failure and pneumonia, rather than surgical procedures, such as joint replacement surgeries and scheduled cardiovascular procedures. Available data from AHRQ's 2006 Healthcare Cost and Utilization Project[47] show all 20 of the most-prevalent diagnosis-related groups (DRG)[48] associated with admissions from the emergency department in 2006 were for medical conditions rather than surgical procedures. In contrast, 7 of the 20 most- prevalent DRGs for nonemergency department admissions in 2006 were for surgical conditions. Officials from the Society for Academic Emergency Medicine told us that because treating surgical conditions is considered more profitable for a hospital than treating emergency medical conditions, hospitals had an incentive to reserve beds for scheduled surgical admissions rather than to give them to patients admitted from the emergency department.[49]

Table 6. Number of Articles Reviewed That Reported Factors Contributing to Emergency Department Crowding

Factor	Number of articles reporting this factor as one of a number of factors contributing to crowding
Lack of access to inpatient beds	45
Lack of access to primary care	22
Shortage of available on-call specialists	7
Difficulty transferring, admitting, or discharging psychiatric patients	3
Other factors[a]	15
Total number of articles reporting factors contributing to emergency department crowding	77

Source: GAO analysis of articles published on or between January 1, 2003, and August 31, 2008.

Notes: Numbers do not sum to total because some articles reported more than one factor.

[a] Five other factors—an aging population, increasing acuity of patients, staff shortages, hospital processes, and financial factors—were mentioned in 15 articles. During our interviews with officials and individual subject-matter experts, however, there was little mentioned about these factors and how they contribute to crowding.

Additional Factors Reported as Contributing to Crowding

Available information suggests that other factors also contribute to emergency department crowding including a lack of access to primary care, a shortage of available on-call specialists, and difficulties transferring, admitting, or discharging psychiatric patients.

Lack of Access to Primary Care

Twenty-two articles we reviewed reported a lack of access to primary care as a factor contributing to emergency department crowding. For example, one of these articles reported that difficulty in receiving care from a primary care provider was associated with an increase in nonurgent emergency department use.[50] Another article described a study in New Jersey that indicated that almost one-half of all emergency department visits within the state that did not result in hospital admission could have been avoided with improved access to primary care services.[51]

Additionally, officials from the Center for Studying Health System Change and the Society for Academic Emergency Medicine mentioned a lack of access to primary care as a factor contributing to emergency department crowding. When patients do not have a primary care physician, or cannot obtain an appointment with a primary care physician, they may go to the emergency department to seek primary care services. In addition, patients who do not have access to primary care may defer care until their condition has worsened, potentially increasing the emergency department resources needed to treat the patient's condition. These situations involve patients that could have been treated outside of the emergency department and may add to the number of patients seeking care at the emergency department.

Articles we reviewed provided conflicting information on the effect of increasing numbers of uninsured patients on emergency department crowding. Five of the 22 articles that mentioned a lack of access to primary care as a factor also reported that increasing numbers of uninsured patients also contributed to emergency department crowding. For example, 1 article indicated that a reason for longer wait times at 30 California hospitals in lower-income areas was that these hospitals treat a disproportionate number of uninsured patients who may lack access to primary care.[52] Two other articles we reviewed, however, suggested that increasing numbers of uninsured patients is not a factor contributing to crowding. For example, the Center for Studying Health System Change reported that contrary to the popular belief that uninsured people are the major cause of increased emergency department use, insured Americans accounted for most of the 16 percent increase in visits between 1996 through 1997 and 2000 through 2001.[53] In addition, officials from AHRQ noted that a larger proportion of patients using the emergency department are insured than uninsured.

Shortage of Available On-Call Specialists

Seven articles and officials from the Center for Studying Health System Change, ACEP, the American Hospital Association, and the American Medical Association whom we interviewed reported that a shortage of on- call specialists available to emergency departments is a factor that contributes to emergency department crowding. Hospitals often employ on-call specialists, meaning specialists such as neurosurgeons or orthopedic surgeons who only travel to the hospital or emergency department when needed and called. When patients wait for long periods in the emergency department for an on-call specialist who is not immediately available—for example, busy covering other hospitals or in surgery—these patients might not receive timely and appropriate care. In addition, these patients may utilize treatment spaces and resources that could be used to treat other patients, potentially crowding the emergency department.

In 2006 IOM reported that over the preceding several years, hospitals had found it increasingly difficult to secure specialists for their emergency department patients.[54] Additionally, another article reported the results of a 2007 American Hospital Association survey of hospital chief executive officers that asked about maintaining on-call specialist coverage for the emergency department.[55] While this survey had a low response rate, it indicates that hundreds of emergency departments reported experiencing difficulty in maintaining on-call coverage for certain specialists. For example, of those chief executive officers that responded to the survey (840 chief executive officers; 17 percent of those surveyed), 44 and 43 percent noted difficulty in maintaining emergency department on-call coverage for orthopedic surgeons and neurosurgeons, respectively. Additionally, officials from the Center for Studying Health System Change told us that delays in obtaining specialty services may contribute to crowding. None of the articles we reviewed, nor officials or individual subject-matter experts we interviewed, quantitatively assessed the relationship between the availability of on-call specialists and emergency department crowding.

Difficulties in Transferring, Admitting, or Discharging Psychiatric Patients

Three articles we reviewed and officials from NCHS, ACEP, and the Center for Studying Health System Change whom we interviewed reported difficulties transferring, admitting, or discharging psychiatric patients from the emergency department as a factor contributing to emergency department crowding. One of these articles reported the results of a national ACEP survey of emergency physicians that asked about psychiatric patients in the emergency department.[56] Of the physicians responding to the survey (328 physicians; approximately 23 percent of those surveyed), about 40 percent reported that, on average, psychiatric patients waited in the emergency department for an inpatient bed longer than 8 hours after the decision to admit them had been made, including about 9 percent who reported that psychiatric patients waited more than 24 hours. Medical patients in the emergency department—those diagnosed with nonpsychiatric conditions—generally waited less time for an inpatient bed: 7 percent of responding physicians reported that, on average, medical patients waited longer than 8 hours after the decision to admit them had been made; slightly less than 1 percent reported that the medical patients waited more than 24 hours. In addition, the survey respondents indicated psychiatric patients waiting to be transferred or discharged added to the burden of an already crowded emergency department and affected access for all patients requiring care. Also, officials from NCHS said that psychiatric patients in the emergency department are a national concern because they are frequent visitors to the emergency department and they may spend more than 24 hours in an emergency department.

National data from NCHS show that, in 2006, psychiatric patients constituted a small percentage of emergency department visits but had a longer average length of stay in the emergency department. Almost 3 percent of emergency department visits in 2006 were by patients presenting with a complaint of a psychological or mental disorder and these patients had an average length of stay in the emergency department that was longer than the average length of stay for all other visits (397 minutes, compared to 194 minutes for all other visits).[57] Emergency department patients with psychiatric disorders may need to be isolated from other patients and may require resources that are not available in many hospitals. Hospital emergency departments often have limited or no specialized psychiatric facilities and emergency department staff may experience difficulties transferring such patients to other facilities, admitting them to the hospital, or discharging them from the emergency department. Additionally, emergency department staff may spend a disproportionate amount of time and resources caring for psychiatric patients while these patients wait for transfer, admission, or discharge.

Other Possible Factors That Contribute to Crowding

Our literature review identified five other factors that may contribute to emergency department crowding. For example, in 2006 IOM reported these five factors—an aging population, increasing acuity of patients, staff shortages, hospital processes, and financial factors—as possible factors that might contribute to emergency department crowding,[58] and these five factors were also mentioned in 14 other articles we reviewed. However, during our interviews with officials and individual subject-matter experts, there was little mentioned about these factors and how they contribute to crowding.

APPENDIX I. SCOPE AND METHODOLOGY

To examine national data made available since 2003 on emergency department diversion and wait times, we obtained and reviewed data collected by the National Center for Health Statistics (NCHS) through its National Hospital Ambulatory Medical Care Survey (NHAMCS).[59] We analyzed available NCHS data[60] for 2001 through 2006 on diversion[61] and wait times[62] to determine what changes, if any, have occurred over time. We analyzed wait time data by patient acuity level[63] and hospital characteristics, such as hospital ownership,[64] metropolitan or nonmetropolitan area location,[65] and geographic region.[66] We analyzed wait times in the emergency department using NCHS's data on recommended time for a patient to see a physician based on patient acuity levels. Further, to determine the average length of stay in the emergency department for patients who presented with a psychological or mental disorder, we analyzed emergency department length of stay by the type of patient complaint at time of the visit. We also analyzed NCHS data on emergency department utilization by payer source, including Medicare, Medicaid, and the State Children's Health Insurance Program,[67] self pay, no charge or charity care; and by hospital characteristics, such as whether the hospital was located in a metropolitan or nonmetroplitan area, to provide context for our work. We also reviewed and analyzed data from the Agency for Healthcare Research and Quality's (AHRQ) Healthcare Cost and Utilization Project[68] to determine the diagnosis-related groups (DRG)[69] most commonly associated with hospital admissions from the emergency department and most commonly associated with non-emergency department admissions—information we determined was related to factors that contribute to crowding.[70] We obtained NCHS and AHRQ data beginning with 2001 because these data became publicly available in 2003 or later, meeting the criterion for inclusion in our analysis. Some data were not available from NCHS for all years between 2001 and 2006 because of revisions made by NCHS to questions on surveys used to collect information and because of low response rates to certain questions on these surveys. At the time we conducted our analysis, the most recent year for which data were available from NCHS and AHRQ was 2006. In this chapter, we present NCHS estimates; for those cases in which we report an increase or other comparison of these estimates, NCHS tested the differences and found them statistically significant.[71] To assess the reliability of national data from NCHS and AHRQ, we interviewed agency officials and reviewed the methods they used for collecting and reporting these data. We resolved discrepancies we found between the data provided to us and data in published reports by corresponding with officials from NCHS to obtain sufficient explanations for the differences.[72] Based on these steps, we determined that these data were sufficiently reliable for our purposes.

To examine information available since 2003 about three indicators of emergency department crowding and the factors that contribute to crowding, we conducted a literature review. In examining information made available since 2003 about indicators and factors of crowding during our literature review, we analyzed articles for what was reported on the effect of crowding on patient quality of care and proposed strategies to address crowding. We conducted a structured search of 16 databases that included peer-reviewed journal articles and other periodicals to capture articles published on or between January 1, 2003, and August 31, 2008. We searched these databases for articles with key words in their title or abstract related to emergency department crowding, or indicators and factors of crowding, such as versions of the word "crowding," "emergency department," "diversion," "wait time," and "boarding." We also included articles published on or between January 1, 2003, and August 31, 2008, that were identified as a result of our interviews with federal officials, professional and research organizations, and subject-matter experts. We also searched related Web sites for additional emergency department crowding publications, including articles reporting on surveys conducted by professional organizations, such as the American Hospital Association. For these articles, we identified the number of respondents and response rates, and for those with lower response rates, we noted them in our report. From all of these sources, we identified over 300 articles, publications and reports (which we call articles) published from January 1, 2003, through August 31, 2008. Within the more than 300 articles, we excluded articles that were published outside of the United States, reported on subjects or data from outside the United States, were only available in an abstract form, had a focus other than day-to-day emergency department operations, or were unrelated to emergency department crowding. We supplemented the articles that were not excluded from our search by reviewing references contained in the bibliography of these articles for additional articles published on or between January 1, 2003, and August 31, 2008, on emergency department crowding that met our inclusion criteria. In total, we included 197 articles[73] in our literature review and analyzed these articles to summarize information on emergency department crowding, including information on diversion, wait times, and boarding, the effect of these indicators of crowding on quality of care, proposed strategies to decrease these indicators, and factors that contributed to emergency department crowding. To review a complete bibliography of these articles, see GAO-09-348SP.

Additionally, we interviewed officials from federal agencies and one state agency, officials from professional, research, and other hospital-related organizations, and individual subject-matter experts to obtain and review information on indicators of emergency department crowding and factors that contribute to crowding. During our interviews, we asked about the effect of crowding on patient quality of care and proposed strategies for addressing crowding. We interviewed federal officials from the Department of Health and Human Services' Centers for Medicare & Medicaid Services and the Office of the Assistant Secretary for Preparedness and Response, and officials from NCHS and AHRQ who have conducted research on emergency department utilization and crowding. We also interviewed officials from the Massachusetts Department of Public Health to discuss the state's planned implementation of a new diversion policy in January 2009. We interviewed officials from professional organizations, including the American College of Emergency Physicians (ACEP), the American Hospital Association, the American Medical Association, the Emergency Nurses Association, the National Association of EMS Physicians, and the Society for Academic Emergency Medicine. Some officials from ACEP and the Society for Academic Emergency Medicine have published research in peer-reviewed journals. In addition, we interviewed officials from research organizations, such as the California Healthcare Foundation, the Center for Studying Health System Change,[74] the Heritage Foundation, and the Robert Wood Johnson

Foundation's Urgent Matters. We interviewed officials from the Joint Commission (an organization involved in hospital accreditation), the Medicare Payment Advisory Commission (an organization that studies Medicare payment issues and reports to Congress), and the National Quality Forum (an organization that develops quality measures for emergency department care). We also interviewed three individual subject-matter experts who have conducted research on emergency department crowding and strategies to reduce crowding.

We conducted this performance audit from May 2008 through April 2009 in accordance with generally accepted government auditing standards. Those standards require that we plan and perform the audit to obtain sufficient, appropriate evidence to provide a reasonable basis for our findings and conclusions based on our audit objectives. We believe that the evidence obtained provides a reasonable basis for our findings and conclusions based on our audit objectives.

APPENDIX II. EMERGENCY DEPARTMENT UTILIZATION, 2001 THROUGH 2006

This appendix provides information on nationally-representative estimates of emergency departments and emergency department visits in the United States by characteristics such as patient acuity level, payer source, hospital ownership type, geographic region, and type of area (metropolitan or nonmetropolitan) from the National Center for Health Statistics' (NCHS) National Hospital Ambulatory Medical Care Survey (NHAMCS). Specifically, for 2001 through 2006[75] this appendix presents the following information:

- the percentage of emergency departments by hospital ownership type, by geographic region, and by type of area (metropolitan or nonmetropolitan) (table 7);
- the number and percentage of emergency department visits by acuity level (figure 5) and payer source (table 8);
- the number and percentage of emergency department visits by hospital
  ownership type, geographic region, and type of area (table 9); and
- the number and percentage of emergency department visits that resulted in hospital admissions (table 10).

Table 7. Percentage of Emergency Departments by Hospital Ownership Type, Geographic Region, and Type of Area in 2001 through 2006

	2001	2002	2003	2004	2005	2006
Hospital ownership type						
Voluntary, nonprofit	62	65	62	67	68	68
Government[a]	27	22	27	25	22	22
Proprietary	11	13	12	8	9	10
Geographic region[b]						
Northeast	15	15	16	15	15	14
Midwest	30	29	29	30	31	29
South	37	38	39	37	37	39
West	18	18	17	18	17	19
Type of area						
Metropolitan[c]	62	60	58	66	65	66
Nonmetropolitan[c]	38	40	42	34	35	34

Source: GAO analysis of NCHS data.

Notes: Percentages may not sum to 100 because of rounding.

[a] NCHS defines a government-owned hospital as a hospital operated by a state, county, city, city- county, or hospital district or authority.

[b] NCHS categorizes geographic regions in the NHAMCS as Northeast, Midwest, South, and West as defined by the U.S. Census Bureau.

[c] *Metropolitan* describes hospitals identified by NCHS as located in a metropolitan statistical area, and *nonmetropolitan* describes hospitals identified by NCHS as not located in a metropolitan statistical area.

Number in thousands (percentage)						
Acuity level[a] (recommended time frame)	**2001**	**2002**	**2003**	**2004**	**2005**	**2006**
Immediate[b] (less than 1 minute)	20,691(19)	24,551(22)	17,297 (15)	14,202 (13)	6,385 (6)	6,084 (5)
Emergent[b] (1 to 14 minutes)					11,313 (10)	12,817 (11)
Urgent (15 to 60 minutes)	34,057 (32)	37,639 (34)	40,128 (35)	41,624 (38)	38,433 (33)	43,666 (37)
Semiurgent (greater than 1 hour to 2 hours)	17,543 (16)	20,427 (19)	22,830 (20)	24,012 (22)	23,870 (21)	26,173 (22)
Nonurgent (greater than 2 hours to 24 hours)	9,790 (9)	11,209 (10)	14,571 (13)	13,774 (13)	16,068 (14)	14,478 (12)
No triaged[c,d]	25,409 (24)	16,328 (15)	19,077 (17)	16,605 (15)	2,397 (2)	1,860 (2)
Unknown[d]					16,857 (15)	14,114 (12)

Source: GAO analysis of NCHS data.

Notes: Percentages may not sum to 100 because of rounding.

[a] NCHS developed time-based acuity levels based on a five-level severity index recommended by the Emergency Nurses Association. The acuity levels describe the recommended amount of time a patient should wait to be seen by a physician.

[b] NCHS added an immediate wait time category to the NHAMCS survey starting in 2005. For 2001 through 2004, the emergent category was defined as a visit with a recommended wait time of less than 15 minutes.

[c] A visit in which there is no mention of an acuity rating or triage level in the medical record, the hospital did not perform triage, or the patient was dead on arrival.

[d] For 2001 through 2004, the NHAMCS survey instrument grouped no triage and unknown triage level into a single category.

Figure 5. Number and Percentage of Emergency Department Visits by Acuity Level in 2001 through 2006

Table 8. Number and Percentage of Emergency Department Visits by Payer Source in 2001 through 2006

Number in thousands (percentage)						
Payer source[a]	**2001**	**2002**	**2003**	**2004**	**2005**	**2006**
Private insurance	43,213 (40)	42,802 (39)	41,461 (36)	39,344(36)	39,565 (34)	40,037 (34)
Medicare	15,879 (15)	16,964 (15)	18,525 (16)	16,909 (15)	16,043 (14)	16,780 (14)
Medicaid/State Children's Health Insurance Program	18,789 (18)	21,751 (20)	24,415 (21)	24,489 (22)	28,661 (25)	30,351 (26)
Worker's compensation	2,665 (3)	2,148 (2)	2,130 (2)	1,964 (2)	1,941 (2)	2,045 (2)
Self-pay[b]	15,854 (15)	15,935 (14)	16,066 (14)	17,669 (16)	18,581 (16)	19,260 (16)
No charge/Charity[b]	1,042 (1)	1,155 (1)	1,113 (1)	885 (1)	885 (1)	1,756 (1)
Other	2,327 (2)	2,551 (2)	2,800 (2)	3,081 (3)	2,184 (2)	3,311 (3)
Unknown	6,024 (6)	5,266 (5)	6,014 (5)	4,946 (4)	5,996 (5)	4,314 (4)
Blank	1,697 (2)	1,582 (1)	1,377 (1)	930 (1)	1,466 (1)	1,337 (1)

Source: GAO analysis of NCHS data.

Notes: Percentages may not sum to 100 because of rounding.

[a] In 2001 through 2004, the survey asked for primary expected source of payment. In 2005 and 2006, multiple sources could be reported. For the purposes of comparability, in

this table, 2005 and 2006 data were recoded to produce a primary expected source of payment based on this hierarchy of responses: Medicare, Medicaid, private insurance, worker's compensation, self-pay, no charge, other, and unknown.

[b] NCHS defines no insurance as having only self-pay, no charge, or charity as payment sources.

Table 9. Number and Percentage of Emergency Department Visits by Hospital Ownership Type, Geographic Region, and Type of Area in 2001 through 2006

Number in thousands (percentage)						
	2001	2002	2003	2004	2005	2006
Hospital ownership type						
	2001	2002	2003	2004	2005	2006
Voluntary, nonprofit	78,458 (73)	76,869 (70)	82,170 (72)	82,117 (75)	83,288 (72)	86,731 (73)
Government[a]	18,663 (17)	20,279 (18)	21,116 (19)	18,832 (17)	19,576 (17)	20,882 (18)
Proprietary	10,370 (10)	13,007 (12)	10,617 (9)	9,267 (8)	12,459 (11)	11,578 (10)
Geographic region[b]						
Northeast	20,802 (19)	18,895 (17)	23,814 (21)	22,274 (20)	22,245 (19)	22,669 (19)
Midwest	26,688 (25)	26,006 (24)	25,205 (22)	26,806 (24)	28,771 (25)	25,735 (22)
South	40,512 (38)	45,544 (41)	44,958 (40)	41,150 (37)	43,871 (38)	50,642 (43)
West	19,489 (18)	19,710 (18)	19,926 (18)	19,986 (18)	20,436 (18)	20,145 (17)
Type of area						
Metropolitan[c]	88,605 (82)	89,170 (81)	92,847 (82)	94,826 (86)	98,622 (86)	100,727 (85)
Nonmetropolitan[c]	18,885 (18)	20,985 (19)	21,056 (19)	15,391 (14)	16,700 (15)	18,464 (16)

Source: GAO analysis of NCHS data.

Notes: Percentages may not sum to 100 because of rounding.

[a] NCHS defines a government-owned hospital as a hospital operated by a state, county, city, city- county, or hospital district or authority.

[b] NCHS categorizes geographic regions in the NHAMCS as Northeast, Midwest, South, and West as defined by the U.S. Census Bureau.

[c] *Metropolitan* describes hospitals identified by NCHS as located in a metropolitan statistical area, and *nonmetropolitan* describes hospitals identified by NCHS as not located in a metropolitan statistical area.

Table 10. Number and Percentage of Emergency Department Visits That Resulted in Hospital Admissions in 2001 through 2006

In thousands						
	2001	**2002**	**2003**	**2004**	**2005**	**2006**
Number of emergency department visits resulting in hospital admissions	12,626	13,471	15,809	14,615	13,867	15,210
Percentage of all emergency department visits resulting in hospital admissions	11.7	12.2	13.9	13.3	12.0	12.8

Source: GAO analysis of NCHS data.

Appendix III. Proposed Measures of Emergency Department Crowding

Researchers continue to use diversion, wait times (including patients who left before a medical evaluation), and boarding as indicators to point to situations in which crowding is likely occurring in emergency departments; however, as we reported in our 2003 report, there is no standard measure of the extent to which emergency departments are experiencing crowding. In the absence of a widely-accepted standard measure of crowding, researchers have proposed and conducted limited testing of potential measures of crowding. During our literature review of articles on emergency department crowding published on or between January 1, 2003, and August 31, 2008, we identified proposed measures of crowding that researchers have tested, either in a single hospital setting or for a limited period of time. Table 11 describes these proposed measures. While researchers have claimed varying levels of success using these measures to gauge crowding, we found no widely accepted measure of emergency department crowding, and that none of these measures of crowding had been widely implemented by researchers and health care practitioners.

Table 11. Proposed Measures of Emergency Department Crowding

Measure	Description	Scale
Emergency department occupancy rate	The total number of patients in the emergency department divided by the total number of licensed emergency department treatment bays available per hour.	An emergency department occu-pancy rate above 1.0 indicates that there are more patients in the emergency department than treatment bays. The higher the emergency department occupancy rate, the more crowded the emergency department.[a]
Emergency depar-tment work index, also known as EDWIN	A summary statistic that descr-ibes the ratio of patients in the emergency department at each triage level compared to the number of attending physicians and unoccupied beds in the emergency department.	Higher EDWIN scores are associated with more crowding in the emergency department, greater acuity among emergency department patients, or both.[b]
Emergency department work score	A composite score that measures where emergency departments utilize resources. The emergency department work score incorpo-rates the number of patients in the waiting room, workload per nurse for patients under evaluation in the emergency department, and the number of patients boarding in the emergency department.	Increases in the emergency department work score indicate an increased probability that an emergency department will go on diversion.[c]
National emer-gency department overcrowding	A screening tool used to deter-mine the degree of emergency department crowding at an	The NEDOCS score is measured on a scale between 0 and 200. Scores over 100 reflect a

Table 11. (Continued)

Measure	Description	Scale
study, also known as NEDOCS	academic institution. NEDOCS incorporates the number of patie-nts in the emergency department, wait times, staffing in the emerg-ency department, and emergency department hours on diversion.	progressively more crowded emergency department.[d]
Real-time emerg-ency analysis of demand indicators, also known as READI	A measure used to predict emergency department demand. The READI analysis evaluates treatment space availability, the acuity of emergency department patients, the productivity of physicians, and an overall measure of demand. The READI analysis uses a bed ratio, an acuity ratio, and a provider ratio to create a demand value score.	Demand value scores greater than 7 should alert the staff to look at each specific ratio to determine possible contributors to demand in excess of emergency department capacity.[e]
Emergency department crowding scale	The scale is used to provide an objective measure of emergency department crowding based on a small set of easily accessible factors. These factors include the number of attending emergency physicians, number of staffed emergency department beds, number of critical-care patients, total number of emergency department patients, number of staffed hospital beds, and hospital occupancy rate.	An emergency department crowding scale score greater than 65 may be predictive of both ambulance diversion and the number of patients who leave without being seen by a physician.[f]

Source: GAO analysis of articles published between January 1, 2003, and August 31, 2008.

[a] M. L. McCarthy, et al., "The Emergency Department Occupancy Rate: A Simple Measure of Emergency Department Crowding?" *Annals of Emergency Medicine*, vol. 51, no. 1 (2008).

[b] S. L. Bernstein, et al., "Development and Validation of a New Index to Measure Emergency Department Crowding," *Academic Emergency Medicine*, vol. 10, no. 9 (2003).
[c] S. Epstein and L. Tian, "Development of an Emergency Department Work Score to Predict Ambulance Diversion," *Academic Emergency Medicine*, vol. 13, no. 4 (2006).
[d] S. Weiss, et al., "Estimating the Degree of Emergency Department Overcrowding in Academic Medical Centers: Results of the National ED Overcrowding Study (NEDOCS)," *Academic Emergency Medicine*, vol. 11, no. 1 (2004).
[e] T. Reeder, et. al ., "The Overcrowded Emergency Department: A Comparison of Staff Perceptions," *Academic Emergency Medicine*, vol. 10, no. 10 (2003).
[f] S. Jones, et al., "An Independent Evaluation of Four Quantitative Emergency Department Crowding Scales," *Academic Emergency Medicine*, vol. 13, no. 11 (2006).

APPENDIX IV. EMERGENCY DEPARTMENT WAIT TIMES

This appendix provides information on nationally-representative estimates of intervals of emergency department wait times in the United States: wait time to see a physician, length of stay in the emergency department, and the percentage of visits in which patients left before a medical evaluation.[76] Specifically, this appendix presents the following information from the National Center for Health Statistics' (NCHS) National Hospital Ambulatory Medical Care Survey (NHAMCS):

- for 2003 through 2006 (the only years for which data were available from NCHS), the percentage of emergency department visits by wait time to see a physician (table 12), average and median wait times to see a physician by patient acuity level (figure 6), average wait times to see a physician by payer type, hospital type, and geographic region (table 13), and average wait times by the hospitals' percentage of visits in which patients left before a medical evaluation (table 14); and
- for 2001 through 2006, the percentage of visits by emergency department length of stay (table 15), the average and median length of stay by patient acuity level (figure 7), the average length of stay in the emergency department by payer type, hospital type, and geographic region (table 16); and average length of stay by the hospitals' percentage of visits in which patients left before a medical evaluation (table 17).

Acuity level[a] (recommended time frame)	2003		2004		2005		2006	
	Avg (SE)[b]	Median	Avg (SE)[b]	Median	Avg (SE)[b]	Median	Avg (SE)[b]	Median
Immediate[c] (less than 1 minute)	23 (2)	12	26 (2)	13	30 (4)	10	28 (3)	11
Emergent[c] (1 to 14 minutes)					36 (3)	15	37 (3)	17
Urgent (15 to 60 minutes)	42 (2)	26	43 (2)	28	55 (2)	32	50 (2)	30
Semiurgent (greater than 1 hour to 2 hours)	60 (2)	42	60 (2)	41	69 (3)	45	68 (3)	45
Nonurgent (greater than 2 hours to 24 hours)	69 (5)	44	65 (3)	42	66 (3)	41	76 (6)	44
No triage[d,e]	48 (5)	25	49 (4)	28	31 (7)	15	45 (6)	22
Unknown[e]					63 (7)	27	66 (11)	30
All Acuity Levels	46 (2)	27	47 (1)	29	56 (2)	31	56 (2)	31

Source: GAO analysis of NCHS data.

Figure 6. Average and Median Wait Time to See a Physician, in Minutes, by Acuity Level, in 2003 through 2006

[a] NCHS developed time-based acuity levels based on a five-level severity index recommended by the Emergency Nurses Association. The acuity levels describe the recommended amount of time a patient should wait to be seen by a physician.

[b] *Avg* is the estimated mean and SE is the standard error of the estimate. Standard error is a statistic used to calculate the range of values that express the possible difference between the sample estimate and the actual population value.

[c] NCHS added an immediate wait time category to the NHAMCS survey instrument starting in 2005. For 2003 and 2004, the emergent category was defined as any visit with a recommended wait time of less than 15 minutes.

[d] No triage indicates a visit in which there is no mention of an acuity rating or triage level in the medical record, the hospital did not perform triage, or the patient was dead on arrival.

[e] For 2003 and 2004, the NHAMCS survey instrument grouped no triage and unknown triage level into a single category.

Table 12. Percentage of Emergency Department Visits by Wait Time to See a Physician, in 2003 through 2006

Wait time to see a physician	2003	2004	2005	2006
Less than 15 minutes	23.4	21.5	22.2	21.9
15 to 59 minutes	39.2	42.3	41.0	39.9
1 hour or more, but fewer than 2 hours	13.3	14.3	15.4	14.8
2 hours or more, but fewer than 3 hours	4.3	4.4	5.2	5.5
3 hours or more, but fewer than 4 hours	1.6	1.8	2.3	2.2
4 hours or more, but fewer than 6 hours	1.4	1.2	1.4	1.4
6 hours or more	0.1	0.1	1.1	0.9
Blank	16.7	14.4	11.4	13.5

Source: GAO analysis of NCHS data.

Note: Percentages may not sum to 100 because of rounding.

Table 13. Average Wait Time to See a Physician, in Minutes, by Payer Type, Hospital Type, and Geographic Region, in 2003 through 2006

	2003 (SE)[a]	2004 (SE)[a]	2005 (SE)[a]	2006 (SE)[a]
Average wait time to see a physician by payer type[b]				
Private insurance	45 (2)	46 (1)	55 (2)	55 (3)
Medicare	40 (2)	43 (1)	52 (3)	52 (3)
Medicaid/State Children's Health Insurance Program	49 (2)	50 (2)	59 (2)	56 (2)
Worker's compensation	37 (3)	46 (2)	39 (3)	41 (3)
Self-pay	50 (2)	49 (2)	57 (3)	62 (4)
No charge/charity	104 (30)	72 (8)	69 (7)	81 (15)
Other	52 (6)	48 (5)	58 (4)	48 (6)
Unknown or blank	48 (3)	56 (4)	64 (3)	57 (5)
Average wait time to see a physician by hospital type				
Voluntary, nonprofit	46 (2)	47 (2)	57 (2)	55 (2)
Government[c]	51 (6)	50 (4)	51 (4)	59 (7)
Proprietary	42 (5)	45 (3)	57 (7)	58 (11)
Average wait time to see a physician by geographic region[d]				
Northeast	48 (3)	51 (3)	57 (4)	56 (3)
Midwest	42 (2)	42 (4)	49 (3)	50 (4)
South	48 (4)	48 (2)	58 (3)	61 (4)
West	48 (5)	50 (3)	63 (6)	49 (5)

Source: GAO analysis of NCHS data.

[a] Average is the estimated mean and SE is the standard error of the estimate. Standard error is a statistic used to calculate the range of values that express the possible difference between the sample estimate and the actual population value.

[b] In 2003 and 2004, the survey asked for primary expected source of payment. In 2005 and 2006, multiple sources could be reported. For the purposes of comparability, in this table, 2005 and 2006 data were recoded to produce a primary expected source of payment based on this hierarchy of responses: Medicare, Medicaid, private insurance, worker's compensation, self-pay, no charge, other, and unknown.

[c] NCHS defines a government-owned hospital as a hospital operated by a state, county, city, city- county, or hospital district or authority.

[d] NCHS categorizes geographic regions in the NHAMCS as Northeast, Midwest, South, and West as defined by the U.S. Census Bureau.

<table>
<tr><th rowspan="2">Acuity level[a] (recommended time frame)</th><th colspan="2">2001</th><th colspan="2">2002</th><th colspan="2">2003</th><th colspan="2">2004</th><th colspan="2">2005</th><th colspan="2">2006</th></tr>
<tr><th colspan="2">Avg (SE)[b] Med[c]</th><th colspan="2">Avg (SE)[b] Med[c]</th><th colspan="2">Avg (SE)[b] Med[c]</th><th colspan="2">Avg (SE)[b] Med[c]</th><th colspan="2">Avg (SE)[b] Med[c]</th><th colspan="2">Avg (SE)[b] Med[c]</th></tr>
<tr><td>Immediate[d] (less than 1 minute)</td><td rowspan="2">197 (8)</td><td rowspan="2">132</td><td rowspan="2">200 (9)</td><td rowspan="2">139</td><td rowspan="2">221 (11)</td><td rowspan="2">149</td><td rowspan="2">228 (11)</td><td rowspan="2">155</td><td>211 (14)</td><td>143</td><td>238 (12)</td><td>174</td></tr>
<tr><td>Emergent[d] (1 to 14 minutes)</td><td>225 (9)</td><td>163</td><td>224 (10)</td><td>168</td></tr>
<tr><td>Urgent(15 to 60 minutes)</td><td>185 (5)</td><td>128</td><td>191 (7)</td><td>133</td><td>201 (7)</td><td>142</td><td>198 (6)</td><td>143</td><td>208 (6)</td><td>153</td><td>204 (6)</td><td>160</td></tr>
<tr><td>Semiurgent (greater than 1 hour to 2 hours)</td><td>163 (4)</td><td>124</td><td>183 (8)</td><td>129</td><td>185 (6)</td><td>134</td><td>184 (6)</td><td>129</td><td>188 (6)</td><td>140</td><td>181 (7)</td><td>136</td></tr>
<tr><td>Nonurgent (greater than 2 hours to 24 hours)</td><td>147 (6)</td><td>108</td><td>155 (7)</td><td>112</td><td>156 (7)</td><td>114</td><td>158 (7)</td><td>115</td><td>161 (5)</td><td>115</td><td>169 (9)</td><td>123</td></tr>
<tr><td>No triage[e,f]</td><td rowspan="2">176 (12)</td><td rowspan="2">115</td><td rowspan="2">216 (23)</td><td rowspan="2">134</td><td rowspan="2">190 (12)</td><td rowspan="2">131</td><td rowspan="2">191 (9)</td><td rowspan="2">133</td><td>123 (8)</td><td>92</td><td>159 (17)</td><td>101</td></tr>
<tr><td>Unknown[f]</td><td>197 (9)</td><td>139</td><td>220 (28)</td><td>141</td></tr>
</table>

Source: GAO analysis of NCHS data.

Figure 7. Average and Median Length of Stay in the Emergency Department, in Minutes, by Acuity Level, in 2001 through 2006

[a] NCHS developed time-based acuity levels based on a five-level severity index recommended by the Emergency Nurses Association. The acuity levels describe the recommended amount of time a patient should wait to be seen by a physician.

[b] *Avg* is the estimated mean and SE is the standard error of the estimate. Standard error is a statistic used to calculate the range of values that express the possible difference between the sample estimate and the actual population value.

[c] *Med* indicates the median measurement.

[d] NCHS added an immediate wait time category to the NHAMCS survey instrument starting in 2005. For 2001 through 2004, the emergent category was defined as a visit with a recommended wait time of less than 15 minutes.

[e] A visit in which there is no mention of an acuity rating or triage level in the medical record, the hospital did not perform triage, or the patient was dead on arrival.

[f] For 2001 through 2004, the NHAMCS survey instrument grouped no triage and unknown triage level into a single category.

Table 14. Average Wait Time to See a Physician, in Minutes, by Hospitals' Percentage of Visits in Which Patients Left before a Medical Evaluation, in 2003 through 2006

Percentage of visits in which patients left before a medical evaluation[a]	2003 Avg (SE)[b]	2004 Avg (SE)[b]	2005 Avg (SE)[b]	2006[c] Avg (SE)[b]
Less than 1 percent	30 (2)	30 (1)	38 (3)	37 (3)
1 percent to 2.49 percent	37 (3)	43 (3)	44 (4)	44 (3)
2.5 percent to 4.49 percent	49 (4)	60 (4)	58 (6)	60 (5)
4.5 percent or more	66 (5)	63 (4)	80 (7)	84 (8)

Source: GAO analysis of NCHS data.

[a] NCHS defines the percentage of visits in which patients left before a medical evaluation as the percentage of visits in which the patient left after triage but before receiving any medical care.

[b] *Avg* is the estimated mean and SE is the standard error of the estimate. Standard error is a statistic used to calculate the range of values that express the possible difference between the sample estimate and the actual population value.

[c] These 2006 data exclude outlier data from a single hospital because a majority of visits to this hospital's emergency department resulted in lengths of stay that exceeded 24 hours.

Table 15. Percentage of Visits by Emergency Department Length of Stay, in 2001 through 2006

Emergency department length of stay	2001	2002	2003	2004	2005	2006
Less than 60 minutes	16.6	15.8	14.0	13.9	13.7	12.8
1 hour or more, but fewer than 2 hours	25.1	25.5	25.2	25.2	24.8	24.0
2 hours or more, but fewer than 4 hours	28.5	30.4	30.9	31.0	31.5	33.0
4 hours or more, but fewer than 6 hours	9.1	10.8	11.5	11.7	12.8	13.9
6 hours or more, but fewer than 10 hours	4.2	5.2	5.7	6.0	6.9	7.3
10 hours or more, but fewer than 14 hours	1.5	1.4	1.4	1.4	1.9	1.7
14 hours or more, but fewer than 24 hours	1.5	1.4	1.4	1.3	1.6	1.0
24 or more hours	0.4	0.8	0.6	0.6	0.2	0.5
Blank	13.4	8.7	9.4	9.0	6.7	5.7

Source: GAO analysis of NCHS data.

Note: Percentages may not sum to 100 because of rounding.

Table 16. Average Length of Stay in the Emergency Department, in Minutes, by Payer Type, Hospital Type, and Geographic Region, in 2001 through 2006

	2001 (SE)[a]	2002 (SE)[a]	2003 (SE)[a]	2004 (SE)[a]	2005 (SE)[a]	2006 (SE)[a]
Average length of stay in the emergency department by payer type[b]						
Private insurance	169 (5)	182 (6)	183 (5)	179 (3)	186 (4)	190 (6)
Medicare	225 (6)	246 (11)	244 (10)	242 (9)	240 (7)	242 (7)
Medicaid/State Children's Health Insurance Program	171 (5)	172 (6)	176 (6)	183 (6)	188 (7)	188 (5)
Worker's compensation	116 (5)	130 (10)	132 (8)	128 (6)	115 (7)	131 (6)

Table 16. (Continued)

	2001 (SE)[a]	2002 (SE)[a]	2003 (SE)[a]	2004 (SE)[a]	2005 (SE)[a]	2006 (SE)[a]
Self-pay	172 (6)	184 (8)	187 (7)	192 (6)	192 (6)	197 (7)
No charge/charity	223 (12)	274 (19)	267 (20)	279 (29)	257 (16)	247 (19)
Other	191 (12)	230 (33)	198 (11)	196 (19)	194 (11)	207 (17)
Unknown	179 (11)	187 (12)	201 (11)	195 (11)	205 (9)	212 (12)
Average length of stay in the emergency department by hospital type						
Voluntary, nonprofit	177 (5)	193 (7)	193 (5)	189 (4)	198 (4)	195 (5)
Government[c]	183 (10)	194 (13)	189 (14)	216 (16)	189 (12)	205 (13)
Proprietary	175 (13)	172 (16)	195 (17)	176 (16)	191 (12)	218 (33)
Average length of stay in the emergency department by geographic region[d]						
Northeast	209 (8)	203 (7)	213 (8)	200 (5)	208 (5)	203 (5)
Midwest	157 (9)	180 (11)	174 (6)	190 (8)	184 (7)	185 (11)
South	173 (6)	184 (7)	191 (9)	186 (6)	189 (7)	206 (10)
West	187 (11)	209 (20)	201 (13)	201 (10)	213 (12)	196 (8)

Source: GAO analysis of NCHS data.

[a] Average is the estimated mean and SE is the standard error of the estimate. Standard error is a statistic used to calculate the range of values that express the possible difference between the sample estimate and the actual population value.

[b] In 2001 through 2004, the survey asked for primary expected source of payment. In 2005 and 2006, multiple sources could be reported. For the purposes of comparability, in this table, 2005 and 2006 data were recoded to produce a primary expected source of payment based on this hierarchy of responses: Medicare, Medicaid, private insurance, worker's compensation, self-pay, no charge, other, and unknown.

[c] NCHS defines a government-owned hospital as a hospital operated by a state, county, city, city- county, or hospital district or authority.

[d] NCHS categorizes geographic regions in the NHAMCS as Northeast, Midwest, South, and West as defined by the U.S. Census Bureau.

Table 17. Average Length of Stay in the Emergency Department, in Minutes, by Hospitals' Percentage of Visits in Which Patients Left Before a Medical Evaluation, in 2001 through 2006

Percentage of visits in which patients left before a medical evaluation[a]	2001 (SE)[b]	2002 (SE)[b]	2003 (SE)[b]	2004 (SE)[b]	2005 (SE)[b]	2006[c] (SE)[b]
Less than 1 percent	137 (7)	150 (12)	147 (6)	152 (6)	145 (6)	150 (8)
1 percent to 2.49 percent	157 (6)	158 (8)	168 (9)	154 (7)	163 (7)	163 (7)
2.5 percent to 4.49 percent	194 (15)	192 (15)	180 (13)	197 (11)	187 (13)	193 (11)
4.5 percent or more	227 (16)	209 (12)	233 (16)	216 (12)	228 (10)	249 (16)

Source: GAO analysis of NCHS data.

[a] NCHS defines the percentage of visits in which patients left before a medical evaluation as the percentage of visits in which the patient left after triage but before receiving any medical care.

[b] Average is the estimated mean and SE is the standard error of the estimate. Standard error is a statistic used to calculate the range of values that express the possible difference between the sample estimate and the actual population value.

[c] These 2006 data exclude outlier data from a single hospital because a majority of visits to this hospital's emergency department had lengths of stay that exceeded 24 hours.

Appendix V. Comments from the Department of Health and Human Services

Note: Page numbers in the draft report may differ from those in this chapter.

DEPARTMENT OF HEALTH & HUMAN SERVICES   OFFICE OF THE SECRETARY

Assistant Secretary for Legislation
Washington, DC 20201

APR 8 2009

Marcia Crosse
Director, Health Care
U.S. Government Accountability Office
441 G Street N.W.
Washington, DC 20548

Dear Ms. Crosse:

Enclosed are comments on the U.S. Government Accountability Office's (GAO) report entitled: Hospital Emergency Departments: Crowding Continues to Occur and Some Patients Wait Longer Than Recommended Time Frames (GAO-09-347) and Special Publication-Hospital Emergency Department: Bibliography (GAO-09-348SP).

The Department appreciates the opportunity to review this report before its publication.

Sincerely,

Barbara Pisaro Clark

Barbara Pisaro Clark
Acting Assistant Secretary for Legislation

Attachment

GENERAL COMMENTS OF THE DEPARTMENT OF HEALTH AND HUMAN SERVICES (HHS) ON THE GOVERNMENT ACCOUNTABILITY OFFICE'S (GAO) DRAFT REPORT ENTITLED: HOSPITAL EMERGENCY DEPARTMENTS: CROWDING CONTINUES TO OCCUR AND SOME PATIENTS WAIT LONGER THAN RECOMMENDED TIME FRAMES (GAO-09-347)

The Department appreciates the opportunity to review and comment on the GAO Draft Report and Special Publication entitled, "Hospital Emergency Departments: Crowding Continues to Occur and Some Patients Wait Longer Than Recommended Time Frames" (GAO-09-347) and "Hospital Emergency Department: Bibliography" (GAO-09-348SP), respectively.

The GAO report, an update of a 2003 GAO survey of the extent of emergency department (ED) crowding, demonstrates that ED waiting times are continuing to increase and frequently exceed national standards; particularly at the highest acuity levels, where delays make the biggest difference. Strengths of the report include its clarity, focus, and a dispassionate tone.

However, designed as an update, it excluded articles and studies published before 2003. This method presupposes that readers will be familiar with the GAO's earlier survey and the large body of literature presented in it. The valid interpretation of this updated information would be strengthened by the content and context of the findings and literature that was reviewed prior to 2003. Moreover, the exclusion of studies conducted outside the US (such as relevant studies conducted in Australia, the UK, and Canada) may limit the readers' insight to this important topic.

Further, the GAO study focuses on the ED and three commonly cited measures of Crowding. It is worth noting that these are process metrics and are limited to patient flow within the Emergency Department. This is potentially important in that they do not provide a direct measure of broader systematic issues of hospital throughput that effect emergency department patient flow such as smoothing elective surgery schedules and facilitating inpatient discharges and bed turnover. Additionally, information regarding process may not be directly related to actual patient outcomes such as treatment success or failure, adverse outcomes or direct harms resulting from the lack of system capacity. The report does discuss this issue on page 19 under "Impact of Crowding" and notes the lack of sufficient quantitative evidence to confirm this assumption, however it may worth specifically noting the limitations of these three process metrics.

End Notes

[1] S. R. Pitts, R. W. Niska, J. Xu, and C. W. Burt, "National Hospital Ambulatory Medical Care Survey: 2006 Emergency Department Summary," *National Health Statistics Reports*, no. 7 (2008).

[2] Medicare is the federal health program that covers seniors aged 65 and older and eligible disabled persons. Medicaid is the joint federal and state program that finances health care for certain low-income individuals. The State Children's Health Insurance Program finances health care for low-income, uninsured children whose family incomes exceed the eligibility limits under their state's Medicaid program.

[3] GAO, *Hospital Emergency Departments: Crowded Conditions Vary among Hospitals and Communities*, GAO-03-460 (Washington, D.C.: Mar. 14, 2003).

[4] We reported, for example, that two out of three metropolitan hospitals reported going on ambulance diversion—that is, asking ambulances to bypass their emergency departments and instead transport patients to other facilities.

[5] The objectives of this committee, the Committee on the Future of Emergency Care in the United States Health System, were to (1) examine the emergency care system in the United States; (2) explore its strengths, limitations, and future challenges; (3) describe a desired vision for the system; and (4) recommend strategies for achieving this vision. The results of the committee's efforts were described in three IOM reports released in 2006: *Hospital- Based Emergency Care: At the Breaking Point*; *Emergency Care for Children: Growing Pains*; and *Emergency Medical Services: At the Crossroads*.

[6] In this chapter, we use the broader indicator *wait times* to include patients leaving before a medical evaluation and intervals of wait times, such as the amount of time patients wait to see a physician and the total time patients spend in the emergency department. The National Center for Health Statistics (NCHS) defines the percentage of visits in which patients left before a medical evaluation as the percentage of visits in which the patient left after triage but before receiving any medical care.

[7] NCHS is an agency within HHS's Centers for Disease Control and Prevention that compiles statistical information to guide actions and policies to improve health. NCHS annually collects data on hospital emergency department utilization in the United States using a nationally representative survey, the National Hospital Ambulatory Medical Care Survey (NHAMCS). NCHS uses the NHAMCS to gather, analyze, and disseminate information on visits to emergency and outpatient departments of nonfederal, short-stay, and general hospitals in the United States. NCHS weights sample data from the NHAMCS to produce national estimates.

[8] AHRQ is an HHS agency that conducts and supports health services research. AHRQ sponsors the Healthcare Cost and Utilization Project, which is a family of health care databases and related software tools and products developed through a federal-stateindustry partnership. Data we reviewed from AHRQ came from the Nationwide Inpatient Sample, which is one of a number of databases and software tools AHRQ developed as part of the Healthcare Cost and Utilization Project.

[9] NCHS uses patient acuity levels to measure a patient's severity of illness. NCHS developed time-based acuity levels based on a five-level emergency severity index recommended by the Emergency Nurses Association. The NHAMCS collects data on five levels of acuity: immediate, emergent, urgent, semiurgent, and nonurgent. Acuity levels are assigned by medical staff after patients arrive in a hospital's emergency department.

[10] I n addition, for those cases in which we present averages based on NCHS data, we are presenting the estimated mean as well as the standard error of the estimate. Standard error is a statistic used to calculate the range of values that expresses the possible difference between the sample estimate and the actual population value.

[11] For the literature review, we included articles reporting results of quantitative analysis, commentaries, articles reporting on literature reviews, or other articles, which includes articles published on or between January 1, 2003, and August 31, 2008, that were identified as a result of our interviews with officials and individual subject-matter experts, and from searches of related Web sites. Other articles include articles that were published by professional associations with reports of their surveys.

[12] NCHS estimates the number of hospitals with an emergency department that is staffed and operated 24 hours a day.

[13] For the purpose of this chapter, we use the term *metropolitan area* to indicate facilities and visits identified by NCHS as occurring in a metropolitan statistical area as defined by the Office of Management and Budget, and *nonmetropolitan area* to indicate facilities and visits identified by NCHS as not in a metropolitan statistical area. The Office of Management and Budget defines a metropolitan statistical area as an area containing a core-based statistical area associated with at least one urbanized area that has a population of at least 50,000, plus adjacent counties having a high degree of social and economic integration with the core as measured through commuting ties with counties contained in the core.

[14] Expected sources of payment on the NHAMCS include private insurance, Medicaid or State Children's Health Insurance Program, Medicare, self-pay, no charge or charity, worker's compensation, other sources, and unknown sources.

[15] NCHS defines uninsured patients as those with expected sources of payment categories of only self-pay, no charge, or charity.

[16] Federal law requires hospitals that participate in Medicare to screen all people and treat any with emergency medical conditions regardless of ability to pay. In certain circumstances, hospitals can place themselves on diversionary status and direct certain en route ambulances to other hospitals when they are unable to accept additional patients.

[17] While researchers have been using diversion, wait times (including patients leaving before a medical evaluation), and boarding as indicators that point to situations in which crowding is likely occurring, there is still no standard measure to quantify the extent to which emergency departments are experiencing crowded conditions. In the absence of a widely-accepted standard measure of crowding, researchers have proposed and conducted limited testing of potential measures of crowding. None of these measures of crowding, however, have been widely implemented by researchers and health care practitioners. See app. III for additional information on these potential measures.

[18] NCHS defines the percentage of visits in which patients left before a medical evaluation as the percentage of visits in which the patient left after triage but before receiving any medical care.

[19] See, B. R. Asplin et al., "A Conceptual Model of Emergency Department Crowding," *Annals of Emergency Medicine*, vol. 42, no. 2 (2003): 173-180.

[20] The average hours spent on diversion in 2003 was 276 hours with a standard error of 42. The average hours spent on diversion in 2006 was 473 hours with a standard error of 73. Standard error is a statistic used to calculate the range of values that expresses the possible difference between the sample estimate and the actual population value.

[21] Diversion data were missing for 3.75 percent of emergency departments in 2003, for 24.1 percent in 2004, for 29.1 percent in 2005, and for 20.5 percent in 2006.

[22] For 2005 and 2006 the sample sizes were insufficient to calculate the average number of hours that nonmetropolitan hospitals reported going on diversion. Therefore, we were not able to compare the number of hours metropolitan and nonmetropolitan hospitals reported spending on diversion.

[23] C. W. Burt and L. F. McCaig, "Staffing, Capacity, and Ambulance Diversion in Emergency Departments: United States, 2003-04," *Advance Data From Vital and Health Statistics*, no. 376 (2006).

[24] For 2003 and 2004, 8 percent of all hospitals reported that their state or local laws prohibit diversion. According to NCHS, some hospitals that reported state laws prohibiting diversion also reported diversion hours. NCHS reported that the reasons for this are unknown but could include respondent or key error, allowable diversions within state laws that prohibit only certain types of diversion, change in state law after the diversion reporting period, or other factors. We did not attempt to validate the number of state or local laws that may govern ambulance diversion.

[25] American Hospital Association, "The State of America's Hospitals," *Taking the Pulse, A Chartpack* (Washington, D.C., April 2006), http://www.aha.org/aha/research-and-trends/health-and-hospital-trends/ (accessed June 26, 2008); and American Hospital Association, "The 2007 State of America's Hospitals," *Taking the Pulse,* (Washington, D.C., July 2007), http://www.aha.org/aha/research-and-trends/health-andhospital-trends/2007.html (accessed June 26, 2008).

[26] In its 2006 survey, the American Hospital Association surveyed about 4,900 community hospital chief executive officers and received 1,011 responses, a response rate of 20 percent. Of those hospitals that responded, about 425 hospitals (about 42 percent of respondents) reported going on diversion at least once during the year. In its 2007 survey, the American Hospital Association surveyed about 5,000 community hospital chief executive officers and

received 840 responses, a response rate of 17 percent. Of those hospitals that responded to the survey, about 302 hospitals (about 36 percent of respondents) reported going on diversion at least once during the year.

[27] The Abaris Group, *California Emergency Department Diversion Project, Report One* (Oakland, Calif.: California HealthCare Foundation, March 2007). http://www.caeddiversionproject.com/uploads/CAEDDiversionProjectReportOne3-21-07.pdf (accessed Sept. 4, 2008).

[28] Maryland Health Care Commission, *Use of Maryland Hospital Emergency Departments: An Update and Recommended Strategies to Address Crowding* (Baltimore, Md., January 2007), http://mhcc.maryland.gov/ hospital_services/acute/emergencyroom/ (accessed Sept. 17, 2008).

[29] In California, the total number of hours that hospitals statewide reported being on diversion decreased overall, from almost 300,000 hours in 2003 to less than 200,000 hours in 2006. The number of hours spent on diversion in individual counties, however, varied over these 3 years, with some counties reporting increases and others reporting decreases. In Maryland, the percentage of time hospitals statewide reported being on diversion increased from 2003 to 2006. Hospitals reported that 9.8 percent and 11.5 percent of their total available hours were spent on diversion in 2003 and 2006, respectively.

[30] NCHS did not collect the average wait time to see a physician in 2001 and 2002.

[31] According to NCHS, from 2003 to 2006 the increases in average wait times to see a physician for visits overall and by emergent, urgent, and semiurgent patients were statistically significant.

[32] NCHS defines emergent patients as patients who, based on triage, are recommended to be seen by a physician within 1 to 14 minutes.

[33] For 2003 and 2006 estimates of average wait time to see physicians at metropolitan hospitals the standard errors are within 2 minutes. For 2003 and 2006 estimates of average wait time to see a physician at nonmetropolitan hospitals the standard errors are within 4 minutes.

[34] Institute of Medicine, Future of Emergency Care, *Hospital-Based Emergency Care: At the Breaking Point* (Washington, D.C.: The National Academies Press, 2006).

[35] L. Fryman and L. Murray, “Managing Acute Head Trauma in a Crowded Emergency Department,” *Journal of Emergency Nursing*, vol. 33, no. 3 (2007).

[36] Institute of Medicine, *Hospital-Based Emergency Care*, 154.

[37] American College of Emergency Physicians, *On-call Specialist Coverage in U.S. Emergency Departments* (Irving, Tex., 2006).

[38] Institute of Medicine, *Hospital-Based Emergency Care*, 4.

[39] C. E. Begley et al., “Emergency Department Diversion and Trauma Mortality: Evidence from Houston, Texas,” *The Journal of Trauma, Injury, Infection, and Critical Care*, vol. 57, no. 6 (2004).

[40] J. M. Pines et al., “The Association between Emergency Department Crowding and Hospital Performance on Antibiotic Timing for Pneumonia and Percutaneous Intervention for Myocardial Infarction,” *Academic Emergency Medicine*, vol. 13 no. 8 (2006). The Joint Commission (formerly the Joint Commission on Accreditation of Healthcare Organizations) and the Centers for Medicare & Medicaid Services have published measures of emergency department quality, including the percentage of patients with community- acquired pneumonia that receive antibiotics within 4 hours of presenting at an emergency department.

[41] D. B. Chalfin et al., “Impact of Delayed Transfer of Critically Ill Patients from the Emergency Department to the Intensive Care Unit,” *Critical Care Medicine*, vol. 35, no. 6 (2007).

[42] The National Health Policy Forum is a nonpartisan organization that provides information on health policy issues and works to foster more informed government decision making. It serves primarily senior staff in Congress, the executive branch, and congressional support agencies.

[43] J. Taylor, *Don't Bring Me Your Tired, Your Poor: The Crowded State of America's Emergency Departments* (Washington, D.C.: National Health Policy Forum, 2006).

[44] See for example, American College of Emergency Physicians, *Emergency Department Crowding: High-Impact Solutions* (Irving, Tex., 2008).

[45] No factor other than a lack of inpatient beds was reported in the articles we reviewed as the main factor contributing to crowding. The next factor most commonly reported as one of a number of factors contributing to crowding was a lack of access to primary care, reported in 22 articles.

[46] Institute of Medicine, *Hospital-Based Emergency Care*, 137.

[47] Data we reviewed from AHRQ came from the Nationwide Inpatient Sample, which is one of a number of databases and software tools AHRQ developed as part of the Healthcare Cost and Utilization Project.

[48] The Centers for Medicare & Medicaid Services uses DRGs to establish payment rates for hospitals that provide medical and surgical services to patients with Medicare.

[49] In addition, available data from AHRQ's Healthcare Cost and Utilization Project indicate that the source of payment for admissions from the emergency department differs in some cases from the source of payment for admissions for elective surgeries. For example, for 2006, AHRQ estimates that of hospital admissions from the emergency department, the source of payment was private insurance for 25 percent of admissions, Medicare for 49 percent of admissions, Medicaid for 15 percent of admissions, uninsured for 8 percent of admissions, and other sources for 4 percent of admissions. In the same year, AHRQ estimates that of hospital admissions for elective surgeries, the source of payment was private insurance for 46 percent of admissions, Medicare for 32 percent of admissions, Medicaid for 15 percent of admissions, uninsured for 3 percent of admissions, and other sources for 4 percent of admissions.

[50] D. C. Brousseau et al., "The Effect of Prior Interactions with a Primary Care Provider on Nonurgent Pediatric Emergency Department Use," *Archives of Pediatric & Adolescent Medicine*, vol. 158, no. 1 (2004).

[51] D. DeLia, *Potentially Avoidable Use of Hospital Emergency Departments in New Jersey* (New Brunswick, N.J.: Rutgers Center for State Health Policy, 2006).

[52] S. Lambe et al., "Waiting Times in California's Emergency Departments," *Annals of Emergency Medicine*, vol. 41, no. 1 (2003).

[53] P. Cunningham and J. May, "Insured Americans Drive Surge in Emergency Department Visits," *Issue Brief*, no. 70 (Washington, D.C.: Center for Studying Health System Change, October 2003).

[54] Institute of Medicine, *Hospital-Based Emergency Care*, 218.

[55] American Hospital Association, "The 2007 State of America's Hospitals," *Taking the Pulse* (Washington, D.C., July 2007), http://www.aha.org/aha/research-and-trends/ (accessed June 26, 2008).

[56] American College of Emergency Physicians, *ACEP Psychiatric and Substance Abuse Survey 2008* (Dallas, Tex., 2008).

[57] The standard error is within 80 minutes for average length of stay in the emergency department for patients presenting with a complaint of a psychological or mental disorder in 2006. The standard error is within 4 minutes for average length of stay in the emergency department for all other patients in 2006.

[58] Institute of Medicine, *Hospital-Based Emergency Care*, 39, 56, 129, 137.

[59] NCHS annually collects national health statistical information on hospital emergency department utilization in the United States using a nationally representative survey, the NHAMCS. NCHS uses the NHAMCS to gather, analyze, and disseminate information on visits to emergency and outpatient departments of nonfederal, short-stay, and general hospitals in the United States. A complex, multistage sample design is used in the NHAMCS, which includes primary sampling units (geographic areas such as counties or groups of counties), hospitals within these units, clinics within outpatient departments, and

patient visits within emergency departments and clinics. Sample data are weighted to produce national estimates. The scope of the emergency department component of the NHAMCS includes emergency departments that are staffed and operated 24 hours a day.

[60] The data provided by NCHS were estimates. Each estimate has a standard error associated with it. For the purposes of this chapter, we report standard errors for averages.

[61] NCHS began collecting data on diversion in a supplement to the NHAMCS that covered the 2-year period of 2003 through 2004. Beginning in 2005, NCHS included a question about diversion on the NHAMCS. Due to the low response rates for the NHAMCS questions about diversion in 2004, 2005, and 2006, we were unable to analyze diversion by characteristics such as hospital type or geographic region. For 2005 and 2006 the sample sizes were insufficient to calculate the number of hours that nonmetropolitan hospitals reported being on diversion. Therefore, we were not able to compare the number of hours metropolitan and nonmetropolitan hospitals reported spending on diversion for those years.

[62] NCHS did not collect data on wait times to see a physician in 2001 or 2002.

[63] To measure severity of illness, NCHS developed time-based acuity levels based on a five- level severity index recommended by the Emergency Nurses Association. The acuity levels describe the recommended amount of time a patient should wait to be seen by a physician. In the 2006 NHAMCS, NCHS collected data on five levels of acuity: immediate, emergent, urgent, semiurgent, and nonurgent.

[64] NCHS uses voluntary nonprofit, government, and proprietary to distinguish hospital ownership. NCHS defines a government-owned hospital as a hospital operated by a state, county, city, city-county, or hospital district or authority.

[65] For the purpose of this chapter, we use the term *metropolitan area* to indicate facilities and visits identified by NCHS as occurring in a metropolitan statistical area as defined by the Office of Management and Budget, and *nonmetropolitan area* to indicate facilities and visits identified by NCHS as not in a metropolitan statistical area. The Office of Management and Budget defines a metropolitan statistical area as an area containing a core-based statistical area associated with at least one urbanized area that has a population of at least 50,000, plus adjacent counties having a high degree of social and economic integration with the core as measured through commuting ties with counties contained in the core.

[66] NCHS categorizes geographic regions in the NHAMCS as Northeast, Midwest, South, and West as defined by the U.S. Census Bureau.

[67] Medicare is the federal health program that covers seniors aged 65 and older and eligible disabled persons. Medicaid is the joint federal and state program that finances health care for certain low-income individuals. The State Children's Health Insurance Program finances health care for low-income, uninsured children whose family incomes exceed the eligibility limits under their state's Medicaid program.

[68] AHRQ sponsors the Healthcare Cost and Utilization Project, which is a family of health care databases and related software tools and products developed through a federal-stateindustry partnership. The Healthcare Cost and Utilization Project databases bring together the data-collection efforts of state data organizations, hospital associations, private data organizations, and the federal government to create a national information resource of patient-level health care data. Data we reviewed from AHRQ came from the Nationwide Inpatient Sample, which is one of a number of databases and software tools AHRQ developed as part of the Healthcare Cost and Utilization Project.

[69] The Centers for Medicare & Medicaid Services uses DRGs to establish payment rates for hospitals that provide medical and surgical services to Medicare beneficiaries.

[70] We also analyzed data from AHRQ's Healthcare Cost and Utilization Project on the source of payment for hospital admissions from the emergency department and admissions not from the emergency department in 2006.

[71] In addition, for those cases in which we present averages based on NCHS data, we are presenting the estimated mean and as well as the standard error of the estimate. Standard

error is a statistic used to calculate the range of values that expresses the possible difference between the sample estimate and the actual population value.

[72] For example, we compared data on the estimated number of emergency departments operating in the United States in 2006 from NCHS with the number of emergency departments operating in the United States in 2006 from the American Hospital Association and found differences. We discussed the discrepancy with NCHS officials and, because we chose in this chapter to use other NCHS estimates, we used NCHS's estimates of the number of emergency departments throughout the report.

[73] For the literature review, we included articles reporting results of quantitative analysis, commentaries, articles reporting on literature reviews, or other articles, including those identified as a result of our interviews with officials and individual subject-matter experts, and from searches of related Web sites. In total, we reviewed 80 articles reporting on quantitative analysis, 64 commentaries, 8 articles reporting on literature reviews, and 45 other articles.

[74] Officials at the Center for Studying Health System Change are researchers who interviewed providers from across the country.

[75] We obtained NCHS data beginning with 2001 because these data became publicly available in 2003 or later, meeting the criterion for inclusion in our analysis. At the time we conducted our analysis, the most recent year for which data were available from NCHS on emergency department utilization was 2006.

[76] The National Center for Health Statistics (NCHS) defines the percentage of patients who left before a medical evaluation as the percentage of visits in which the patient left after triage but before receiving any medical care.

In: Issues in Providing Emergency Medical Care ISBN: 978-1-61761-595-5
Editor: Mary E. Mathers

Chapter 3

EMERGENCY RESPONSE: CIVIL LIABILITY OF VOLUNTEER HEALTH PROFESSIONALS

Vivian S. Chu

SUMMARY

The devastation inflicted on the Gulf region by Hurricanes Katrina and Rita in 2005 and Hurricanes Gustav and Ike in 2008, in addition to recent disasters in the Midwest due to tornadoes and flooding, triggered mass relief efforts by local, state, and federal government agencies, as well as private organizations and individuals. As unpaid volunteers have carried out much of the relief effort, some have questioned whether such volunteers—particularly medical personnel, so-called "volunteer health professionals" (VHPs)—will be protected from potential civil liability in carrying out their duties. This chapter provides a general overview of the various federal and state liability protections available to VHPs responding to disasters. This chapter does not discuss liability of VHPs who go abroad to render assistance.

INTRODUCTION

In 2008, various communities across America were hit hard by natural disasters ranging from the great floods in Iowa to tornadoes in the Midwest and Hurricanes Ike and Gustav in the Gulf region. When volunteers go to these disaster areas as they did when Hurricane Katrina hit Louisiana and the surrounding states in 2005, questions arise as to the potential civil liability of those volunteer health professionals (VHPs)—individually licensed medical professionals who gratuitously provide medical services in response to these regions' clear need for medical skills and services. The concern is that the potential threat of medical malpractice liability, in particular, may give pause to these VHPs.

This chapter discusses the patchwork of federal and state laws that operate to protect volunteers generally, which can include VHPs, and those laws that trigger liability protection only for VHPs[1]—with a focus on some of the midwestern states in addition to the Gulf region. Whether a VHP is protected from civil liability depends on a number of factors, including under whose control the VHP operates and whether or not a state of emergency has been declared. The liability protections discussed in this chapter generally shield volunteers from *civil* liability for negligent conduct (i.e., a failure to take adequate care that results in injuries or losses to others). Civil liability for conduct that is more egregious than mere negligence, such as willful, or grossly negligent conduct, is not protected, unless otherwise noted. Criminal conduct is also not protected.

VOLUNTEER PROTECTION ACTS

Laws shielding volunteers from liability have been enacted on both the federal and state level; the statutes discussed in this section apply in non-emergency situations as well as emergency situations. On the federal level, Congress passed the Volunteer Protection Act (VPA) in 1997.[2] This statute provides immunity for ordinary negligence to volunteers (not only medical volunteers) of non-profit organizations or governmental entities so long as (1) the volunteer was acting within the scope of his or her responsibilities; (2) the volunteer was licensed or certified in the state where the harm occurred, *if licensure or certification was required*; (3) the harm was not the result of willful action, grossly negligent behavior, etc.; and (4) the harm was not caused by the volunteer's operation of a vehicle.[3] The act does not prohibit the non-profit or governmental entity from bringing a civil action against its own volunteers, nor does the act shield from liability the non-profit or governmental entity for the actions of its volunteers. Furthermore, the VPA expressly preempts state standards that provide less protection than the act.[4]

All 50 states and the District of Columbia have enacted their own volunteer protection statutes that provide varying degrees of liability protection.[5] These state statutes are not preempted by federal law so long as they provide greater liability protections. Mississippi, for instance, provides broad civil liability protection to any volunteer who qualifies under the statute by providing services *or* goods to a volunteer agency, unless the injury complained of was the result of (a) conduct that was intentional, grossly negligent, etc., or (b) the operation of a motor vehicle.[6] Texas also provides immunity to volunteers of a charitable organization for any act or omission resulting in death, damage, or injury if the volunteer was acting in the course and scope of the volunteer's duties or functions.[7]

Many states, in addition to having VPA-type laws, have enacted statutory provisions geared specifically toward volunteer health professionals (VHPs). These statutes are like VPAs in that they provide immunity from civil liability and are not dependent on, or triggered by, an emergency situation. As discussed above, Texas has statutory provisions that provide immunity to ordinary volunteers of charitable organizations, but it also has an additional statutory provision that shields from civil liability a VHP who serves as a direct service volunteer of a charitable organization.[8] Another example is Oklahoma's Volunteer Medical Professional Services Immunity Act,[9] which protects Oklahoma-licensed VHPs from civil liability, when among other things, such VHPs receive no compensation and the patient signs a consent form. Mississippi similarly protects Mississippi-licensed medical personnel and extends this liability protection to other medical personnel who receive special volunteer licenses to practice in the state.[10] Likewise, Alabama provides civil liability protections to VHPs who gratuitously provide limited medical services as part of an "established free medical clinic." Under Alabama's statute, VHPs can be licensed in any state to receive protection.[11] By contrast, Louisiana's statute that similarly protects licensed VHPs operating as part of nonprofit medical clinics provides no reference as to whether such protection is limited only to those VHPs licensed in Louisiana or whether it includes out-of- state medical licensees. [12]

Good Samaritan Statutes

In addition to VPAs, every state and the District of Columbia has enacted its own "Good Samaritan" statute, which protects from civil liability individuals who gratuitously provide emergency assistance.[13] Generally, Good

Samaritan statutes lower the applicable standard of care owed by the person providing assistance. [14] These statutes were first enacted to protect the doctor, who, although under no duty to help, provides emergency assistance to another but fails to adhere to the otherwise applicable standard of care when doing so. "Emergency" in this context refers to medical emergencies. Many Good Samaritan statutes require that the volunteer or rescuer, in order to be eligible for immunity, act in good faith and must not have received or expected any compensation for his or her efforts.[15] Not all Good Samaritan statutes are the same, as some protect a narrow class of individuals such as physicians and other medically licensed personnel, while others protect a broader class of persons such as the casual bystander who renders emergency assistance.[16] Another example of how Good Samaritan statues vary is that some limit protection to care provided at the scene of an "accident," whereas others apply to an "emergency"; some apply to both accidents and emergencies.[17]

Illinois, Alabama, and Louisiana, for instance, have Good Samaritan laws that offer broad but varying degrees of coverage to medically related personnel. Illinois's Good Samaritan law protects physicians licensed in *any* American state or territory who provide emergency care, so long as the resulting harm was not caused by willful or wanton conduct.[18] Again, however, the term "emergency" is used in the medical context, and courts are left to determine on a case-bycase basis what constitutes an emergency that triggers the act's protections.[19] Alabama's Good Samaritan statute protects medical personnel who gratuitously and in good faith provide emergency care "at the scene of an accident, casualty, or disaster" from *all* civil liability.[20] Louisiana's Good Samaritan statute provides liability protection to medical personnel licensed in Louisiana who provide medical services "at the scene of an emergency."[21] Medical personnel licensed to practice in another state, however, do not enjoy protection under Louisiana's Good Samaritan statute, but they cannot be prosecuted for practicing without a license when they offer gratuitous assistance in an emergency situation.[22] In contrast, Iowa's Good Samaritan statute protects from liability all individuals, not just medical personnel, who render emergency care or assistance "at the place of emergency or accident or while the [injured] person is in transit" unless their acts or omissions constitute reckless or willful and wanton misconduct.[23]

Debate exists as to how far Good Samaritan laws should extend in terms of who is covered and for what kind of actions. In California, for example, there has been much controversy surrounding the California Supreme Court decision in *Van Horn v. Watson*,[24] which held that the state statute only shields rescuers from liability if they provide medical care in an emergency situation.

The *Van Horn* case stems from a 2003 car accident in the Los Angeles area where the passenger- defendant pulled the plaintiff out of what she thought was a smoldering car at risk of exploding.[25] The plaintiff was left a paraplegic and sued Torti, one of the defendants, for negligence. Torti sought immunity under California's general Good Samaritan provision.[26] The court of appeals held and the California Supreme Court affirmed that the civil liability protections did not apply to Torti because she was not providing emergency medical care to the plaintiff. Since the ruling in December 2008, California lawmakers amended the Good Samaritan provision to offer greater legal liability protections to those who "render emergency medical *or nonmedical* care at the scene of an emergency."[27]

EMERGENCY POWERS AND PUBLIC HEALTH EMERGENCY STATUTES

Except insofar as they waive it, the federal and state governments enjoy sovereign immunity from suit.[28] The federal government has waived this immunity with the passage of the Federal Tort Claims Act,[29] and some state governments have similar statutory provisions.[30] Such acts generally immunize government employees from tort liability for torts committed within their scope of employment, and instead allow the government to be held liable in accordance with the law of the state where a tort occurred. Thus, apart from the general VPAs and Good Samaritan statutes, one additional way to shield VHPs from individual civil liability during an emergency is to declare them non-paid employees of the federal government or a state government for liability purposes.[31] This can be done for particular volunteers in all situations or only when a general state of emergency or public health emergency has been declared.[32]

Emergencies can be declared at both federal and state levels by the President of the United States, a state governor, and sometimes by other local authorities.[33] Every state has a regime for declaring a general emergency or disaster, and such a declaration can explicitly trigger liability protections or allow the governor to do so.[34] Kansas's emergency management statute, for example, shields state government employees, agents, and volunteer workers from civil liability for any death or injury to persons or damage to property as a result of any activity performed during the declared emergency, except where there is willful misconduct, bad faith, or gross negligence.[35] In such an emergency situation, Kansas's provisions also deem any member of a regional medical emergency response team to be a state employee for liability purposes.[36] Alabama's statutory provisions protects a broad group of "emergency management workers," as the definition of the term includes employees, volunteers, or entities of *other* states performing emergency management services during a declared emergency.[37] By contrast, Mississippi's emergency management statute provides civil liability protection only to state government employees and agents during a declared emergency.[38]

In addition to general emergency procedures, some states have regimes for public health emergencies, which, like general emergency management statutes, provide varying degrees of coverage.[39] The declaration of a public health emergency triggers special protections for medical personnel, which often includes liability protection for VHPs.[40] Florida's health emergency statute, for example, extends the liability protections that state employees enjoy to all volunteers who respond to a public health emergency declaration.[41] Louisiana's health emergency statute declares that "during a state of public health emergency, any health care providers (licensed instate) shall not be civilly liable for causing the death of, or injury to, any person, or damage to any property except in the event of gross negligence or willful misconduct."[42]

Even where emergency or public health emergency statutes do not explicitly grant liability protections to VHPs, these statutes generally allow governors to impose such protections for volunteers where appropriate. In 2005, for example, Louisiana Governor Kathleen Blanco, pursuant to her public health emergency powers, issued an executive order temporarily suspending all licensure requirements for medical volunteers (so long as they are licensed in other states) and declaring such volunteers to be state employees shielded from civil liability.[43]

EMERGENCY MUTUAL AID AGREEMENTS

Emergency mutual aid agreements may be instituted among political subdivisions and Indian tribal nations within a state, out-of-state with neighboring political subdivisions, or internationally with Canadian provinces. Approved by Congress in 1996, the Emergency Management Assistance Compact (EMAC),[44] which has been codified into state statutes, provides a prearranged structure for a state to request aid from other states when affected by disaster. Since 1996, all fifty states have agreed to the terms of EMAC, as have the District of Columbia, Puerto Rico, the U.S. Virgin Islands, and Guam. In addition to EMAC, states have entered into other interstate mutual aid agreements.[45]

EMAC addresses concerns regarding liability protection and represents an attempt by its signatories to remove legal obstacles that can impede the flow of aid from bordering states in times of emergency. Under EMAC, a person from one state who renders assistance in another and who holds a license, certificate, or other permit for the practice of professional, mechanical, or other skills is considered to be licensed, certified, or permitted to exercise those duties in the requesting state, subject to limitations or conditions set by the governor of the requesting state.[46] Notwithstanding the recognition of out-of-state licenses, reciprocity is not automatically extended to VHPs who do not provide services pursuant to an EMAC request for assistance. Unless authorities can verify an individual's claims, they may be reluctant to accept the individual's professional services, particularly where VHPs arrive "spontaneously."

Verifying whether a VHP is properly licensed during a time of emergency can become problematic. Following the terrorist attacks in 2001, Congress authorized creation of the Emergency System for Advance Registration of Volunteer Health Professionals (ESAR-VHP)[47] so that emergency managers and others could have the ability to quickly identify and facilitate the use of VHPs in local, state, and federal emergency responses.[48] The ESAR-VHP program, which is based in the Office of the Assistant Secretary for Preparedness and Response in the Department of Health and Human Services (HHS), assists state and local authorities by developing standardized state-based programs for registering and verifying the credentials of VHPs in advance of disasters or emergencies.[49] As of August 8, 2008, 40 states and territories had operational ESAR-VHP systems and it was expected that all 50 states would have operational systems by the end of 2008.[50] It also appears that there is movement toward integrating the Medical Reserve Corp, which is housed under the Office of the U.S. Surgeon General, and the ESAR-VHP system.[51]

EMAC also provides that when officers or employees of one state render aid in another, they are treated as agents of the requesting state for tort and immunity purposes.[52] Neither the officers or employees of the state providing assistance, nor that state itself, would face liability for acts or omissions committed in good faith while rendering aid (including providing supplies and related equipment). While EMAC clearly offers liability protections of which

VHPs could avail themselves, these protections may be limited in that they appear to apply only to state officers and employees. However, by entering into agreements with VHPs to extend employee status, home states can extend EMAC liability protection to VHPs.

ACKNOWLEDGMENTS

This chapter was initially written by legislative attorneys Kathleen S. Swendiman and Nathan Brooks.

End Notes

[1] Various commentators have offered suggestions for creating an across the board standard governing VHP liability in disaster situations. *See, e.g.*, James J. Hodge, Jr., Lance A. Gable, and Stephanie H. Calves, *Volunteer Heath Professionals and Emergencies: Assessing and Transforming the Legal Environment*, 3 Biosecurity and Bioterrorism: Biodefense Strategy, Practice and Science 216 (2005) *available at* http://www.liebertonline.com/toc/bsp/3/3.

[2] P.L. 105-19, codified, as amended, at 42 U.S. C. § 14501 *et seq*. For background, *see* CRS Report 97-490, *Volunteer Protection Act of 1997*, by Henry Cohen.

[3] 42 U.S.C. § 14503(a).

[4] *Id*. at § 14503(d). However, the VPA allows states to enact statutes "declaring the election of such [a] State that this Act shall not apply to such civil action in the State." If a state does so, then the VPA would not apply in any action if all parties to the action are citizens of the state. *See id*. at § 14502. Thus far, only New Hampshire has done so.

[5] Sharon Hoffman, *Responders' Responsibility: Liability and Immunity in Public Health Emergencies*, 96 Geo. L.J. 1913, 1944 (2008).

[6] Miss. Code. Ann. § 95-9-1 (2008).

[7] Tex. Civ. Prac. & Rem. § 84.004(a) (2007).

[8] *Id*. at § 84.004(c).

[9] Okla. Stat. tit. 76, § 32 (2008).

[10] Miss. Code. Ann. § 73-25-38(1), (3).

[11] Ala. Code. § 6-5-663 (2008).

[12] La. Rev. Stat. § 9:2799.5(1), (3) (2008).

[13] Stewart R. Reuter, *Physicians as Good Samaritans*, 20 J. Legal Med. 157 (1999).

[14] *Id*. at 158.

[15] Carl V. Nowlin, *Don't Just Stand There: Help Me!*, 30 Wm. Mitchell L. Rev. 1001, 1007 (2004).

[16] *Id*. at 1008.

[17] *Id*.

[18] 745 Ill. Comp. Stat. 49/25 (2008).

[19] See *Rivera v. Arana*, 322 Ill. App. 3d 641, 651 (2001).

[20] Ala. Code. § 6-5-3 32.

[21] La. Rev. Stat. Ann. § 37:1731(A).

[22] *Id*. at § 37:1731(B).

[23] Iowa Code § 613.17 (2008).

[24] 45 Cal. 4th 322 (2008).

[25] Jim Sanders, "Legislature seeks to aid good Samaritans; Bills would expand liability protection for rescue efforts," Sacramento Bee, Jan. 14, 2009, at A1.

[26] Cal. Health & Safety Code § 1799.102. (2008) ("No person who in good faith, and not for compensation, renders emergency care at the scene of an emergency shall be liable for any civil damages resulting from any act or omission.").

[27] Cal. Health & Safety Code § 1799.102 (2009) ("(B)(2) ... no person who in good faith, and not for compensation, renders emergency medical or nonmedical care or assistance at the scene of an emergency shall be liable for civil damages resulting from any act or omission other than an act or omission constituting gross negligence or willful or wanton misconduct.").

[28] Federal sovereign immunity traces its roots to the English common law doctrine that the state can do no wrong. State sovereign immunity appears to derive from the same source, and the Supreme Court has held that the states did not lose this essential power upon ratification of the federal Constitution. *Alden v. Maine*, 527 U.S. 706 (1999).

[29] 28 U.S.C. §§ 1346(b), 2671-80. *See* CRS Report 95-717, *Federal Tort Claims Act (FTCA)*, by Vivian S. Chu.

[30] *See, e.g.*, Fla. Stat. § 768.28 (2008); Tex. Civil Prac. and Remedies Code Ann. § 101.025 (2008); La. Rev. Stat. Ann. § 13:5108.1 (2008).

[31] The Pandemic and All-Hazards Preparedness Act provides an example of such tort liability protections. Under 42 U.S.C. § 300hh-11(d)(1), the Secretary of Health and Human Services may appoint volunteer health professionals as intermittent personnel of the National Disaster Medical System (NDMS), which provides medical services when a disaster overwhelms local emergency services. NDMS volunteers benefit from the same immunity from civil liability as the employees of the Public Health Service. The Secretary may also accept the assistance of the VHPs as temporary volunteers under 42 U.S.C. § 217b. Under applicable regulations, such volunteers may receive legal protections including protection from civil liability claims under the FTCA. *See e.g.*, 45 C.F.R. § 57.5; *see* http://www.hhs.gov/ aspr/opeo/ndms/join/index.html

[32] *See also* CRS Report RS20984, *Public Health Service Act Provisions Providing Immunity from Medical Malpractice Liability*, by Henry Cohen; CRS Report 97-579, *Making Private Entities and Individuals Immune from Tort Liability by Declaring Them Federal Employees*, by Henry Cohen.

[33] *See* Sharona Hoffman, *Responders' Responsibility: Liability and Immunity in Public Health Emergencies*, 96 Geo. L.J, 1913, 1921 (2008).

[34] For a discussion of the federal government's public health emergency preparedness, *see* CRS Report RL33579, *The Public Health and Medical Response to Disasters: Federal Authority and Funding*, by Sarah A. Lister; For a discussion of state public health emergency preparedness, *see* James G. Hodge and Evan D. Anderson, *Principles and Practice of Legal Triage During Public Health Emergencies*, 64 N.Y.U. Ann. Surv. Am. L. 649 (2008), *available at* http://www1.law.nyu.edu/pubs/annualsurvey/issues

[35] Kan. Stat. Ann. §48-9 15 (2008).

[36] *Id.* at § 48-915(c).

[37] Ala. Code. § 3 1-9-16(d).

[38] Miss. Code. Ann. § 33-15-21(a).

[39] For example, Florida has statutory provisions that address both emergency management (Fla. Stat. §§ 252.31 *et seq*) and public health emergencies (Fla. Stat. §§ 381.00315). On a federal level, the Secretary of the Department of Health and Human Services can also declare a public health emergency pursuant to the Public Health Service Act.

[40] The terrorist attacks of September 11, 2001, and the subsequent anthrax scare, spurred states to draft legislation to facilitate widespread health emergencies. At the request of the Centers for Disease Control and Prevention, Professor Lawrence Gostin spearheaded the effort to draft the Model State Emergency Health Powers Act (MSEHPA). Under the Model Act,

VHPs "shall not be liable for any civil damages as a result of medical care or treatment related to the response to the public health emergency." For additional information about the MSEHPA, *see* James G. Hodge, Jr., and Lawrence O. Gostin, *The Model State Emergency Health Powers Act*, January 2002, *available at* http://www.publichealthlaw.net/MSEHPA/Center%20MSEHPA%20Commentary.pdf.

[41] Fla. Stat. § 38.00315(2); 768.28(9)(a).

[42] La. Rev. Stat. Ann. § 29:771(c).

[43] State of Louisiana Executive Department, Executive Order No. KBB 2005-33 (September 12, 2005). It is important to note that licensure of medical professionals is a state matter and that there is no national licensing system. In 2006, Louisiana codified § 29:735.1 that provides immunity to volunteer medical health professionals: "During a declared state of emergency anywhere in the State, any health care provider who in good faith voluntarily renders emergency care or first aid to assist persons as a result of emergency whether the aid is rendered in the area subject to the declaration of emergency or elsewhere shall not be civilly liable for causing death, injury to, or any person or damage to any property except in the event of gross negligence or willful misconduct."

[44] P.L. 104-321, 110 Stat. 3877. EMAC is intended to encourage mutual assistance in "any emergency or disaster that is duly declared by the governor of the affected state(s)," including "natural disaster, technological hazard, man-made disaster, civil emergency aspects of resources shortages, community disorders, or enemy attack." EMAC, Art. I. *See also* CRS Report RL34585, *The Emergency Management Assistance Compact (EMAC): An Overview*, by Bruce R. Lindsay.

[45] For example, several states belong to or authorize forest fire compacts, including Montana, New York, and Wyoming. Other states, like New Jersey and New York, have mutual aid statutes that provide for mutual aid during an enemy attack in order to protect bridges, tunnels, and other major infrastructure components.

[46] EMAC, Art. V.

[47] Public Health Security and Bioterrorism Preparedness and Response Act § 107, 42 U.S.C. § 247d-7b.

[48] Integration of Medical Reserve Corp and the Emergency System for Advanced Registration of Volunteer Health Professionals *available at* http://www.medicalreservecorps.gov/File/ESAR_VHP/ ESAR- VHPMRC IntegrationFactSheet.pdf. As EMAC applies to other non-medically licensed professionals, states may include non-health professional volunteers in their registries. *See id.*

[49] The ESAR-VHP program was initially based in the Health Resources and Services Administration Office upon its creation in 2002. However, Congress moved the program in 2006 when it created the Office of the Assistant Secretary for Preparedness and Response in HHS with the passage of the Pandemic and All-Hazards Preparedness Act, P.L. 109- 417.

[50] Emergency System for Advanced Registration of Volunteer Health Professionals Presentation, MRC Region V Conference by Steve Tise, *available at* http://www.medicalreservecorps.gov/file/MRC_Resources/RegionV/ Regional_Conference_Aug_2008/ESAR-VHP_Tise.pdf. As of February 2010, it is unclear whether all 50 states have an operational ESAR-VHP as expected.

[51] *See* Integration, *supra* note 48. The Medical Reserve Corp (MRC) is a national network of community based volunteer units that assists existing local agencies with public health activities throughout the year, and with preparedness and response activities in times of need. In April 2009, the MRC co-sponsored the 2009 Integrated Medical, Public Health, Preparedness and Response Training Summit with the NDMS, ESAR-VHP, and the Office of Force Readiness and Deployment. However, as of February 2010, the status of integration between MRC and ESARVHP is unclear.

[52] EMAC, Art. VI.

In: Issues in Providing Emergency Medical Care ISBN: 978-1-61761-595-5
Editor: Mary E. Mathers

Chapter 4

PUBLIC HEALTH AND MEDICAL PREPAREDNESS AND RESPONSE: ISSUES IN THE 111TH CONGRESS

Sarah A. Lister

SUMMARY

Key recent events—the 2001 terrorist attacks, Hurricane Katrina, and concerns about an influenza ("flu") pandemic, among others—sharpened congressional interest in the nation's systems to track and respond to public health threats. The 109th Congress passed several laws that established, reorganized, or reauthorized key public health and medical preparedness and response programs in the Departments of Health and Human Services (HHS) and Homeland Security (DHS). The 110th Congress was engaged in oversight of the implementation of these laws, focused in particular on such matters as (1) the fitness of HHS and DHS—in terms of authority, funding, policies, and workforce—to respond to health emergencies; (2) the effectiveness of coordination among them and other federal agencies; and (3) the status of major initiatives such as pandemic flu preparedness and disaster planning for at-risk populations. The 111th Congress is likely to remain engaged in oversight of the nation's readiness for health threats.

The Obama Administration may reconsider homeland security objectives and priorities established by the George W. Bush Administration. Shifts in doctrine or priority, if any, may manifest as key positions are filled, or in the budget proposal for FY2010.

The 111th Congress may review HHS's disaster response capabilities, including its authority to declare a public health emergency and the means to fund its response efforts. Among other things, it is not clear that a flu pandemic would qualify for major disaster assistance under the Robert T. Stafford Disaster Relief and Emergency Assistance Act (the Stafford Act). Also, although the HHS Secretary has authority for a no-year Public Health Emergency Fund, Congress has not appropriated monies to the fund for many years. Finally, since Hurricane Katrina, Congress has urged and HHS has adopted a more aggressive federal role in the response to health emergencies.

Historically, federal assistance to states in dealing with disasters has come mainly as guidance and funding for preparedness and response activities. Since Hurricane Katrina, the federal role has been more direct, involving, for example, more procurement and deployment of medical response assets. Congress may wish to consider whether this trend is appropriate and sustainable.

At this time, there is no federal assistance program designed purposefully to cover the uncompensated or uninsured health care costs for disaster victims. The 111th Congress may reconsider earlier proposals to provide such assistance under certain circumstances.

Health emergencies often involve scarcities of resources (including personnel), movement restrictions, business and school closures, and other constraints. While state and local governments have the primary authority over such measures as quarantine and isolation, a comprehensive response to a public health emergency may involve overlapping governmental authorities and attendant legal and economic issues.

The 108th Congress launched Project BioShield to encourage the development of medical countermeasures. Some concerns remain about the program's ability to attract private-sector developers. Also, the 109th Congress provided a means for liability protection for product developers and others, if countermeasures are used during a health emergency. A program to compensate persons who may be injured by such covered countermeasures has not been funded.

This chapter summarizes key issues in domestic public health and medical preparedness and response, citing other CRS Reports and sources of additional information.

BACKGROUND

Three important principles color the issues in public health and medical preparedness and response. First, preparedness and response are different functions. At each level of government, they involve different leadership roles, legal authorities, organizational structures, and funding mechanisms. Generally, during an incident, certain conditions must be met before a jurisdiction can implement response activities, or access funds reserved for that purpose. Second, states and localities, rather than the federal government, are the seats of authority and responsibility for the oversight of both health care and emergency management. For example, state laws generally authorize governors to order and enforce the evacuation of residents in emergency situations. Except under extraordinary circumstances, the federal government generally does not dictate the conduct of health care or emergency management activities to state or local officials, or to health care providers.[1] Finally, most public health functions—broad, population-based programs, such as restaurant inspections to assure food safety—are inherently governmental. In contrast, the nation's health care system—which delivers professional health care services to individuals—is primarily private and for-profit. Providers and facilities operate in an increasingly competitive marketplace in which emergency planning is not always seen as a necessary expense.

The 2001 terrorist attacks, the flawed response to Hurricane Katrina, and concerns about an influenza ("flu") pandemic sharpened congressional interest in the nation's ability to track and respond to health threats. The 109th Congress established or reauthorized relevant programs and activities in the Departments of Health and Human Services (HHS) and Homeland Security (DHS). The 110th Congress focused on oversight of these activities, in particular (1) the fitness of HHS and DHS—in terms of authority, funding, policies, and workforce—to respond to health emergencies; (2) the effectiveness of federal agency coordination; and (3) the status of major initiatives such as pandemic flu preparedness and disaster planning for at-risk populations.

The 111th Congress is likely to remain engaged in oversight of the nation's readiness for health threats. It faces a different and dynamic landscape, however. The Obama Administration will likely usher in some shifts in preparedness priorities, in direction and degree yet to be shown. The nation's health care system is the subject of a vigorous reform debate. Although emergency management is not the focus of that debate, significant system reforms, if enacted, would likely affect emergency planning needs and system response capacity. And the nation's unsettled economy poses a dilemma for policy makers. Future spending for public programs may be significantly constrained, unless a program were seen as a means for job creation, or some other engine of economic stimulus. It remains to be seen where federal programs to address health emergencies will fit into this complex picture.

This chapter, which will be updated as needed, summarizes key issues in domestic public health and medical preparedness and response, citing other CRS Reports and sources of additional information.

KEY LEGISLATION IN PRIOR CONGRESSES

The 109th Congress enacted two comprehensive laws affecting public health and medical preparedness and response. The Pandemic and All-Hazards Preparedness Act (PAHPA, P.L. 109- 417), passed in 2006, established or extended programs for public health emergency preparedness and response activities in HHS, and established a Biomedical Advanced Research and Development Authority (BARDA) in HHS to oversee the development and procurement of medical countermeasures (e.g., diagnostic tests, drugs, and vaccines).[2] The Post-Katrina Emergency Management Reform Act of 2006 (PKA, Title VI of P.L. 109-29 5) reorganized DHS and, within it, the Federal Emergency Management Agency (FEMA). The PKA also codified the position of DHS Chief Medical Officer, with primary responsibility within DHS for medical issues related to natural and man-made disasters and terrorism.[3]

ISSUES FOR CONGRESS

Government Leadership, Organization, and Capacity

The Presidential Transition

The Obama Administration may reconsider any number of homeland security objectives, and its priorities are likely to differ, at least somewhat, from those of the George W. Bush Administration. For example, the Bush Administration placed considerable emphasis on the detection of and response to a large-scale biological attack. Among other things, it established the

BioWatch system of air monitors in major cities, and redirected federal funds from states to these cities to bolster planning for mass dispensing of antibiotics in response to an attack. These efforts were widely critiqued. Some said they were excessive, draining resources from routine public health and biomedical research needs. Others said they were insufficient to protect the public in a timely manner. Still others questioned the basic effectiveness of the programs. Critiques are likely to continue, whether or not the Obama Administration maintains its predecessors' priorities.

The transition also marks the first transfer of presidential authority for the Department of Homeland Security (DHS), and for a number of homeland security positions and programs established since 2001. These positions include the Assistant Secretary for Health Affairs and Chief Medical Officer at DHS (DHS CMO),[4] the Assistant Secretary for Preparedness and Response (ASPR) in the Department of Health and Human Services (HHS), and their corresponding offices and activities.

Shifts in doctrine or priority in the new Administration, if any, may manifest when key positions are filled, or when the budget proposal for FY20 10 is unveiled.

Executive Branch Organization

The 111th Congress may consider removing FEMA from DHS and re-establishing it as a separate agency, as it was in the Clinton Administration. Other substantial reorganizations of federal homeland security agencies do not appear to be under debate at this time. Congress may consider relocating certain programs, however. (See, for example, the subsequent section "Select Agent Program.") Also, President Obama may consider reorganizing certain homeland security functions, such as those of the Homeland Security Council (HSC). President George W. Bush established the HSC in the Executive Office of the President shortly after the 2001 terrorist attacks.[5] From 2005 through 2008, the HSC served as the hub of federal preparedness activities for pandemic flu, involving HHS, DHS, the State Department, and other federal departments and agencies.[6] Some have called for a merger of the HSC with the larger National Security Council (NSC), citing a number of responsibilities shared by the two.[7] It is reported that President Obama has called for a comprehensive review of the functions of the NSC.[8]

Federal Leadership and Coordination

For public health and medical preparedness and response, the roles and responsibilities of principals in HHS and DHS have shifted in past years. The

109th Congress provided some clarity, but refinement of these roles and responsibilities is likely to continue for some time to come. Pursuant to the PAHPA and the PKA, applicable activities in DHS are led by the DHS CMO, and in HHS by the HHS ASPR. The PKA provided that the DHS CMO "shall have the primary responsibility *within the Department* for medical issues related to natural disasters, acts of terrorism, and other man-made disasters," while the PAHPA provided that the "Secretary of [HHS] shall lead all *Federal* public health and medical response to public health emergencies and incidents.... "[9] (Emphasis added.) Hence, the Secretary of Homeland Security leads all federal emergency and disaster response activities; the DHS CMO leads both preparedness and response activities for public health and medical care, but only within DHS; and the Secretary of HHS, through the ASPR, leads all federal public health and medical response activities, under the overall leadership of the Secretary of Homeland Security.

The Government Accountability Office (GAO) noted, in the context of pandemic flu planning, that " ... these leadership roles involve shared responsibilities, and it is not clear how these would work in practice."[10] GAO recommended that DHS and HHS conduct training and exercises to ensure that federal leadership roles are clearly defined and understood. In February 2009, GAO reported that although some recommended activities have been undertaken, it is unclear whether these exercises rigorously tested federal leadership roles in a pandemic.[11]

Federal incident response activities are coordinated according to the *National Response Framework* (NRF), and "all-hazards" blueprint published by DHS.[12] Public health and medical response activities (under the leadership of HHS) are laid out in an annex called *Emergency Support Function #8*, or ESF-8. These activities, at the federal, state, and local levels, are commonly referred to as ESF-8 activities. The NRF replaced the earlier National Response Plan, incorporating lessons from the flawed response to Hurricane Katrina. Nonetheless, some leadership gaps and conflicts remain in ESF-8. In addition to the inter-related roles of the HHS ASPR and the DHS CMO discussed above, there are concerns about a lack of leadership clarity for responder health and safety (see "The Health and Safety of Disaster Responders"); emergency sheltering; mass fatality management; and mental health services, among others.[13]

On January 28, 2009, DHS Secretary Janet Napolitano announced an action directive to review the Department's plans for the response to a large-scale medical incident. [14] The directive required specific DHS offices and components, working with state and local partners, to review and assess current plans (including ESF-8 in the NRF), relevant homeland security grant programs, and other matters. DHS components were to report to the Secretary by February 24, 2009.

Strategic Planning

The PAHPA requires the HHS Secretary to publish a comprehensive, all-hazards national public health and medical response strategy and implementation plan (the "National Health Security Strategy," or NHSS), beginning in 2009, and quadrennially thereafter. [15] The NHSS is to include a process for achieving a number of preparedness goals enumerated in the statute. In 2007, the Bush Administration published a homeland security directive to establish a "national strategy for public health and medical preparedness," including implementation steps.[16] The directive stated that the principles and actions it contained were to be incorporated into the NHSS, and serve as a foundation to address the preparedness goals prescribed by the PAHPA.

On September 30, 2008, the Office of the HHS ASPR awarded a delivery order (a type of contracting mechanism) to the RAND Corporation, to provide support in developing the NHSS during FY2009.[17] The 111th Congress may be interested in monitoring the NHSS development process, in particular whether the leadership of the Office of the HHS ASPR maintains steady progress toward completion during the Obama Administration, and the extent to which the strategy and its accompanying plans and goals reflect, or are consistent with, any changes in doctrine or priority that may be adopted by the new Administration.

HHS Response Capability and Funding Authority

The 111th Congress may consider the adequacy of permanent authorities of the HHS Secretary for responding to public health threats, including authority to declare a public health emergency and the expanded authorities that flow from it.[18] Members of Congress may also consider how HHS funds any of its disaster response activities that are not reimbursable by FEMA. Although the HHS Secretary has authority for a no-year Public Health Emergency Fund, Congress has not appropriated monies to the fund for many years. Also, it is not clear that a flu pandemic would qualify as a major disaster under the Robert T. Stafford Disaster Relief and Emergency Assistance Act (the Stafford Act). The definition of major disaster in the law does not explicitly include or exclude infectious diseases, and past interpretations of the provision's applicability to bioterrorism and naturally occurring infectious diseases have varied. If major disaster assistance were applicable in a flu pandemic, substantial FEMA funds could be available to support HHS response activities. [19]

State Grants for Public Health and Health System Preparedness

Since 2002, Congress has provided more than $9 billion in grants to states to strengthen public health and hospital preparedness for public health threats. The PAHPA extended the programs, adding authority to withhold funds for failure to meet program requirements, a state matching requirement, and a requirement that the Secretary of HHS publish certain information about program activities and performance on a public website.[20] The Cooperative Agreement for Public Health Emergency Preparedness is administered by the Centers for Disease Control and Prevention (CDC).[21] The Hospital Preparedness Program is administered by the HHS ASPR.[22] The programs have been challenging for federal managers and state awardees alike. Among other things, federal managers have had difficulty developing meaningful and measurable performance goals for the programs.[23] Also, state awardees have had some difficulty staffing their preparedness programs. Some have cited, as explanations, public health workforce shortages, and the challenges of recruiting with annual discretionary or "soft" funding.[24]

Economic Stimulus

In February 2009, Congress passed and the President signed P.L. 111-5, the American Recovery and Reinvestment Act of 2009 (ARRA), a package of spending and tax cuts intended to stimulate the nation's flagging economy. The law provided $50 million for cyber-security improvements at HHS. Earlier versions of the legislation would also have provided (1) $430 million for the advanced development and procurement of medical countermeasures through the Biomedical Advanced Research and Development Authority (BARDA);[25] and (2) $420 million for pandemic flu preparedness for facility construction and the development and/or purchase of vaccines, drugs, supplies, and equipment. The BARDA and pandemic provisions were removed in conference.[26] The law did not include enhanced funding for the CDC or HHS/ASPR public health or hospital preparedness grants to states, discussed earlier.[27]

Health System Preparedness and Response

Medical Surge Capacity

Policymakers have long been concerned about medical surge capacity, that is, the ability of health systems to manage large increases in caseloads that would result from mass casualty incidents. The successful response to such incidents requires the coordination of several elements, which are variously based in federal, state or local authority, or in the private sector. These elements are (1) patients, who may require rescue or medical evacuation; (2) a treatment facility, which may be an existing hospital, or a field tent with cots; (3) a competent health care workforce; (4) medical equipment and non-perishable medical supplies; (5) drugs, vaccines, tests and other perishable medical supplies; (6) a system of medical records; and (7) a health care financing mechanism.

Facing growing cost constraints for several decades, the largely private health care sector has sought to avoid having the unused, reserve capacity (such as empty beds) that would be needed in such situations. Since 2001, the federal government has sought to establish this capacity in the private sector, with mixed success. For example, the HHS Hospital Preparedness Program (described above) makes grants to state governments to work with private health care facilities and systems in assuring regional surge capacity, but the effectiveness of the program has been questioned.[28]

Historically, the federal government has helped states with disaster response primarily by providing guidance and funding for preparedness activities, and assisting with the costs of response activities. During Hurricane Katrina, the shortcomings of this approach with respect to medical surge capacity were evident. Since then there has been an expansion of the federal role through direct procurement and deployment of medical response assets, providing a stronger backstop for state, local, and private-sector response efforts. For example, the PAHPA authorized HHS to acquire mobile medical assets, such as Field Medical Stations (FMS).[29]

HHS assets and personnel were deployed extensively for the evacuation and care of individuals with special needs before and during Hurricanes Gustav and Ike in the Fall of 2008.[30] The Strategic National Stockpile (SNS) of medical supplies and drugs, as well as the National Disaster Medical System and other programs to provide emergency health workers, have also been expanded since 2005.[31] The costs to *procure* FMS and SNS assets are borne in annual discretionary appropriations and may be fairly easily tracked. In contrast, many of the costs to *deploy* these and other assets in a disaster response, in addition to the staffing costs required to support these deployments, are often reimbursed by FEMA from the Disaster Relief Fund.[32] The federal government has not published information about the costs associated with HHS 's responses to Hurricanes Gustav and Ike. The Congress may be interested in seeking information about these costs, in order to determine whether they represent an appropriate and sustainable investment of federal effort.

Finally, the 111th Congress may examine the performance of the federal Crisis Counseling Assistance and Training Program (CCP), which is authorized in the Stafford Act and administered jointly by HHS, FEMA, and the states to address mental health problems among disaster victims.[33] The response to Hurricane Katrina in 2005 prompted a re-examination of the CCP and other federal assistance programs that address disaster mental health. Concerns include the lack of a sound evidence base to identify effective services, the timeliness of services provided, the appropriate scope and duration of these services, and matters of organization, cost, and accountability. For example, the respective roles and responsibilities of HHS (which provides technical expertise for state CCP programs through its Substance Abuse and Mental Health Services Administration), FEMA (which funds the state programs), and states and their contractors (which implement them) are not always clear.

Workforce Surge Capacity

The HHS Health Resources and Services Administration (HRSA) manages several health professions programs intended to alleviate shortages and maldistributions of physicians, nurses, and others who provide health care services to individuals.[34] These programs are not, however, geared toward assuring disaster surge capacity in the health care workforce. Efforts to bolster the ranks of health professionals for disaster response include ensuring civil liability protection for volunteer health professionals, and establishing a national system to verify their licenses and credentials. While efforts are ongoing among states and on the federal level, a uniform system for protection of volunteer health professionals does not yet exist.[35]

Surge capacity in the public health workforce—those workers who assure safe food and water, conduct diseases surveillance, and carry out other public health activities in response to disasters—has received little federal attention until recently. The PAHPA authorized a loan repayment demonstration project for individuals who serve in state or local health departments in defined areas of need, but the authority has not been implemented.[36]

At this time, the National Disaster Medical System, administered by the HHS ASPR,[37] and the Medical Reserve Corps, administered by local governments with the assistance of the HHS Office of the Surgeon General,[38] provide surge capacity to bolster the local disaster response workforce in both health care and public health.

The Health and Safety of Disaster Responders

Responsibility for the health and safety of disaster response workers is a matter of concern in the National Response Framework (NRF). GAO found that the efforts of the Occupational Safety and Health Administration (OSHA, in the Department of Labor) during the response to Hurricane Katrina were hampered by confusion about OSHA's role. GAO noted in particular that disagreements between FEMA and OSHA regarding OSHA's role delayed FEMA's authorization of mission assignments to fund OSHA's response activities.[39] Some Members of Congress and others sought to have worker health and safety elevated from a Support Annex to an Emergency Support Function in the NRF, which would have given OSHA more autonomy in commencing its response activities.[40] Instead, the NRF contains a revised Worker Safety and Health Support Annex.[41]

Disaster Victims and Health Care Costs

There is no federal assistance program designed purposefully to cover the uncompensated or uninsured costs of individual health care that may be needed as a result of a disaster.[42] There is not consensus that this should be a federal responsibility. Nonetheless, if faced with a mass casualty incident, hospitals, physicians, and other providers could face considerable pressure to deliver care without a clear source of reimbursement.

Congress or the Bush Administration provided special assistance to address this concern three times in response to recent disasters. Following the September 11, 2001 terrorist attacks, HHS provided funding to hospitals, clinics, and other health care facilities (including privately owned facilities) near the three affected sites (in NY, PA, and VA), that either provided unreimbursed health care services to victims, or suffered other economic hardship as a result of road closures or other infrastructure effects.[43] Through intermittent appropriations, Congress has funded a program to provide medical screening, monitoring, and treatment services to responders and others who were exposed to hazards at the World Trade Center site in NY following the 2001 terrorist attack, and who are now experiencing health problems that are believed to have resulted from those exposures.[44] Following Hurricane

Katrina, Congress provided $2 billion to cover the state share of Medicaid costs associated with evacuees and individuals living in declared disaster areas (for states with approved federal waivers), and to restore access to care in affected areas.[45]

Legislative proposals in the 110th Congress would have: authorized the HHS Secretary to use a special fund to provide temporary emergency health care coverage for uninsured individuals affected by public health emergencies (H.R. 6569/S. 3312); or addressed the health care needs of responders and others who are ill purportedly as a result of exposures at World Trade Center (WTC) site in NY following the 2001 terrorist attack (for example, H.R. 1414/ S. 201, S. 1119, H.R. 1247, H.R. 3543, H.R. 6594, and H.R. 7174). None of these proposals was enacted. H.R. 847, the James Zadroga 9/11 Health and Compensation Act of 2009, has been introduced in the 111th Congress to address WTC-related illnesses.

Medical Monitoring Following a Disaster

After the 2001 terrorist attack on the World Trade Center, some responders developed chronic health problems believed to have resulted from hazardous exposures during the rescue, recovery, and clean-up operations.[46] Efforts to track and address these problems were hampered because, at the outset, no central registry was established to identify all responders and other on-site workers, and no program was established to monitor their health going forward, in order to quickly detect common or unusual illness patterns in the cohort.

Following Hurricane Katrina, the 109th Congress enacted the SAFE Port Act (P.L. 109-347). One of its provisions authorizes the President, acting through the Secretary of HHS and pursuant to a major disaster declaration under the Stafford Act, to establish medical monitoring programs, if needed, to track the health status of individuals (not limited to responders) who may experience hazardous exposures as a result of the disaster.[47] The authority has not yet been implemented. According to GAO, as of May 2008, HHS had not articulated a plan for doing so.[48] Federal agency responsibilities and funding mechanisms are not clear without such a plan. For example, within HHS, at least three components—the ASPR, as well as the Agency for Toxic Substances and Disease Registry and the National Institute for Occupational Safety and Health, both in CDC—have relevant authorities and responsibilities that overlap. Also, a major disaster typically triggers federal coordinating mechanisms laid out in the NRF, which places OSHA in the lead in assuring responder health and safety.[49] In 2008 GAO recommended, for future disasters, that HHS develop plans to register all responders during a disaster, as part of a comprehensive departmental plan to assure responder health during and after disasters.[50] GAO said that such a plan should also include a means to implement medical monitoring programs, or to assist states and localities in doing so. To meet the intent of the SAFE Port Act, such a plan must also address affected individuals who are not responders.

Planning for the Needs of Special Populations

The terrorist attacks of 2001 and the hurricanes of 2005 showed that some people may be at greater risk, or more in need of special services, during and after a disaster.[51] The PAHPA requires the Secretary of HHS to consider, in emergency planning, the needs of at-risk individuals, defined as children, pregnant women, senior citizens, and others as determined by the Secretary. The PKA required the head of FEMA to appoint a Disability Coordinator, charged, among other things, with coordinating emergency management policies and practices for individuals with disabilities.[52] The 110th Congress authorized and appropriated funds for a National Commission on Children and Disasters, which has been established in the HHS Administration for Children and Families.[53]

The 111th Congress is likely to be interested in the continued evolution of these efforts, in particular, how well these federal efforts address the diversity of special needs that exist in the population, and how well they are coordinated with each other in planning, and during disaster response. GAO has commented, for example, that the Office of the FEMA Disability Coordinator has generally not coordinated its work with a key federal agency—the National Council on Disability—as it is required to do by the PKA.[54]

Defense against Specific Threats

Pandemic Influenza Preparedness

To prepare for the threat of a human flu pandemic, the 109th Congress provided $6.1 billion in emergency supplemental funding for FY2006.[55] Most of it has supported an HHS initiative to expand domestic vaccine production capacity.[56] The Congressional Budget Office (CBO) has analyzed the uncertainties and financial risks associated with this robust investment in applied research and infrastructure development, noting that the success of the

HHS initiative may be affected, among other things, by the outcomes of research efforts to improve vaccine technology, and the extent to which the demand for seasonal flu vaccine can sustain the costs of expanded production capacity and more sophisticated vaccine production technology over the long term.[57] GAO has made a number of recommendations regarding pandemic response planning, coordination, and capacity in recent years, and reported in February 2009 that many of the recommendations had not yet been fully implemented.[58]

Given the considerable federal investment in preparing for this threat, the 111th Congress is likely to remain interested in the status of national preparedness efforts. Additional issues of potential interest may include (1) the priority given by the Obama Administration to continued planning efforts, including its budget request for FY2010; (2) future federal leadership for planning efforts (see the earlier discussion of the HSC in the section "Executive Branch Organization"); and (3) the status of state preparedness efforts.[59] Finally, as mentioned earlier, it is not clear that a flu pandemic would qualify as a major disaster under the Stafford Act.[60] If so, substantial FEMA funds could be made available for HHS response activities. If not, alternative funding options available to the Secretary of HHS are limited. (See the earlier section of this chapter, "HHS Response Capability and Funding Authority.")

Communicable Disease Control

The response to communicable disease threats may involve movement restrictions, business and school closures, compulsory treatments, and other constraints. While state and local governments have the primary authority over these domestic containment measures, a comprehensive response to a public health emergency may involve overlapping governmental authorities and attendant legal and economic issues.[61]

Managing employers' and workers' concerns during outbreaks of communicable disease—in particular, a flu pandemic—may be especially difficult. For example, if workers fear losing their employment or their wages, compliance with public health measures such as isolation or quarantine may suffer. Although public health officials typically recommend, whenever possible, that isolation or quarantine measures be voluntary rather than compulsory, voluntary measures may not provide the same level of job protection for workers who miss work in order to comply with them. [62]

Recent incidents have expanded Congress's longstanding interest in the security of U.S. borders to include concerns about communicable diseases in travelers, which is a matter of federal jurisdiction. These incidents have brought into question the divisions of authority and effectiveness of coordination among federal agencies that are responsible for disease control, and for the security of the borders and the transportation infrastructure.[63] Policy makers have noted that if these systems are unable to respond to common and expected infectious disease threats such as tuberculosis, they may also be unable to respond to more serious threats such as pandemic flu or bioterrorism. Effective solutions are elusive, but would ideally address scientific, technical, and economic constraints; the balance of individual and collective rights; and the roles of federal, state, and local authorities, and foreign governments.

Finally, health emergencies often involve scarcities of resources, including personnel, equipment, drugs, and vaccines. Prioritizing the use of these resources to maximize benefit requires careful study of scientific and medical evidence, and raises complex legal and ethical questions that are best considered before emergencies arise.[64]

Biodefense Laboratory Capacity and Oversight

Since 2001, HHS, DHS, USDA, the Department of Defense (DOD), state governments, and some academic institutions have expanded or are expanding their laboratory capacity to study or test for dangerous biological pathogens and toxins. These laboratories play a key role in the biodefense effort, offering the hope of better responses to a biological attack and a better understanding of the bioterrorism threat. However, they could also increase the risk of a biological attack by being a source of materials or training. In 2008, the congressionally mandated Commission on the Prevention of Weapons of Mass Destruction Proliferation and Terrorism recommended, among other things, the expansion of government oversight of these laboratories.[65]

The 111th Congress may consider issues associated with domestic biodefense laboratories, such as the effectiveness of current oversight efforts, the appropriate balance between security and the transparency that fosters scientific discovery, and possible effects of domestic regulatory approaches on international collaboration.[66] Legislation introduced in the 111th Congress (S. 485/H.R. 1225)[67] would require the HHS Secretary to review and report to Congress regarding, among other things, the adequacy of current and planned laboratory capacity, and information sharing between the biodefense and infectious disease communities. The Secretary would also be required to develop minimal training standards for personnel, and to establish a voluntary reporting system through which laboratory personnel could report accidents and other incidents.

Select Agent Program

Legislation introduced in the 111th Congress (S. 485/H.R. 1225) would reauthorize the Select Agent Program, which is jointly managed by the CDC and the U.S Department of Agriculture (USDA) Animal and Plant Health Inspection Service (APHIS) to regulate certain biological pathogens and toxins that could be used for bioterrorism.[68] Program authority expired at the end of FY2007. The bills would require, among other things, a program review, planning for surges in testing capacity, and guidance to improve inventory practices. They would also authorize HHS and USDA to release certain sensitive information about the program to designated state officials if a state's laws are adequate to protect against the further release of such information. The bills would leave program administration under CDC and APHIS, as it is now.

In August 2008, the Federal Bureau of Investigation (FBI) announced that it believed a DOD scientist had been responsible for the 2001 anthrax attacks.[69] The individual took his own life before charges could be filed, so the case will not reach a legal conclusion. Nonetheless, the incident has heightened concerns about the effectiveness of security risk assessments ("background checks") that FBI conducts on individuals who are registered in the Select Agent Program and granted access to the pathogens. Subsequently, the Commission on the Prevention of Weapons of Mass Destruction Proliferation and Terrorism—which was mandated by Congress before the matter involving the anthrax scientist was publicly known—recommended a comprehensive review of the Select Agent Program.[70]

The Commission did not recommend that leadership for the Select Agent Program be changed. However, at a hearing on the Commission's report, Senators Joseph Lieberman and Susan Collins (the Chairman and Ranking Member, respectively, of the Senate Committee on Homeland Security and Governmental Affairs) signaled that they may introduce legislation to put DHS in charge of regulating biological pathogens.[71] CDC and APHIS have the scientific and technical expertise to support the program, but the Senators were concerned that they may lack the homeland security and national security expertise that is also required. However, some members of the biomedical research community were concerned about proposals to move the program into DHS when legislation to establish the new department was under consideration in 2002.[72] They argued, successfully at the time, that the program should remain with CDC and APHIS.

Development, Procurement, and Use of Countermeasures

Project BioShield

The 108th Congress launched Project BioShield to encourage the development of countermeasures that lack commercial markets. (The program is not limited to procurement of biodefense countermeasures. Products to address radiological, chemical, and other threats are also considered.) DHS and HHS have shared responsibility for the program since its inception, although the process by which procurement decisions are made has changed several times.[73] At this time, DHS manages a 10-year advance appropriation (through FY2013) to purchase countermeasures, and is responsible for conducting *Material Threat Determinations* (MTDs) to assess whether a particular hazard—such as an anthrax or sarin gas attack—poses a threat to national security. In response to an MTD, HHS evaluates the threat, and the potential need for countermeasures, in a public health context. Funds for development and procurement are drawn from the 10-year appropriation, with the approval of the President, following joint recommendations from the Secretaries of HHS and DHS.

The 109th Congress established, in the PAHPA, the Biomedical Advanced Research and Development Authority (BARDA) in HHS to support countermeasure development and facilitate communication between the government and developers. The PAHPA also required the HHS Secretary to develop and publish a strategic plan to guide HHS countermeasures research, development, and procurement.[74]

The BioShield program has experienced numerous problems over the years, and many have been resolved.[75] Key issues that remain are (1) the clarity of the shared roles of DHS and HHS; and (2) whether HHS can define contract terms that are perceived by product developers as sufficiently clear and lucrative to be worth their investment. The first concern appears to have improved over time, partly as a result of successive directives from Congress and the Bush Administration. Given the program's limited history of successful procurements, the second concern may persist and continue to be of interest to the 111th Congress.

Finally, intellectual property protections may affect the availability of countermeasures by making them more commercially attractive to developers, or more costly to purchasers, including governments.[76]

Liability and Compensation

In December 2005, Congress passed Department of Defense Emergency Supplemental Appropriations, 2006 (P.L. 109-148), including Division C, titled the "Public Readiness and Emergency Preparedness Act" (PREP Act). Upon a declaration of emergency, the PREP Act eliminates liability, except in the case of willful misconduct, of manufacturers and others involved in the production, distribution, and use of covered countermeasures. [77] In October 2008, HHS Secretary Leavitt made several such emergency declarations with respect to countermeasures for smallpox, anthrax, botulism, and acute radiation sickness, and amended a prior declaration for pandemic flu countermeasures.[78] Each declaration is in effect through 2016, unless amended.

The law also establishes, in the U.S. Treasury, a "Covered Countermeasure Process Fund" to compensate those who may be harmed by a covered countermeasure. As of FY2009, the fund has not received an appropriation. No funding was requested in the annual budget submissions of the Bush Administration.

Expired Program Authorities

The 111th Congress may consider reauthorization of expired preparedness and response programs.[79] These include authority for HHS health professions programs, which expired in 2002.

These programs, in Title VII of the Public Health Service Act, aim to address underserved areas and populations, and have not focused on emergency preparedness and response in the past. However, the last reauthorization in 1998 preceded heightened concerns regarding this matter since 2001.[80] Also, although authority for the Strategic National Stockpile of countermeasures was amended since the terror attacks of 2001, general program authority expired at the end of FY2006 and has not been extended.[81] In addition, as discussed earlier, authority for the Select Agent program to regulate biological pathogens expired at the end of FY2007.

End Notes

[1] The federal government can, however, attach conditions to the expenditure of federal grant funds, in furtherance of national goals.

[2] CRS Report RL33589, *The Pandemic and All-Hazards Preparedness Act (P.L. 109-417): Provisions and Changes to Preexisting Law*, by Sarah A. Lister and Frank Gottron.

[3] P.L. 109-295, 120 Stat. 1409, 6 U.S.C. § 321e.

[4] In the George W. Bush Administration, one individual served in this position with both titles.

[5] CRS Report RS22840, *Organizing for Homeland Security: The Homeland Security Council Reconsidered*, by Harold C. Relyea. The HSC was subsequently codifed in the Homeland Security Act, P.L. 107-296; 6 U.S.C. § 491 *et seq*.

[6] See, for example, comments of Frances Fragos Townsend, Former Assistant to President George W. Bush for Homeland Security and Counterterrorism, hearing of U.S. Congress, Senate Committee on Homeland Security and Governmental Affairs, *Structuring National Security and Homeland Security at the White House*, 111th Cong., 1st sess., February 12, 2009.

[7] See, for example, Rob Margetta, "Is HSC and its Chief Transitioning Out of the New Administration?," *CQ Homeland Security*, December 3, 2008. For more information about the NSC, see CRS Report RL3 0840, *The National Security Council: An Organizational Assessment*, by Richard A. Best Jr.

[8] Karen DeYoung, "Obama's NSC Will Get New Power," *Washington Post*, February 8, 2009, p. A1.

[9] P.L. 109-295, 120 Stat. 1409; P.L. 109-417, § 101, 120 Stat. 2832.

[10] U.S. Government Accountability Office, *Influenza Pandemic: Opportunities Exist to Clarify Federal Leadership Roles and Improve Pandemic Planning*, GAO-07-1257T, September 26, 2007, http://www.gao.gov; and CRS Report RL33579, *The Public Health and Medical Response to Disasters: Federal Authority and Funding*, by Sarah A. Lister.

[11] U.S. Government Accountability Office, *Influenza Pandemic: Sustaining Focus on the Nation's Planning and Preparedness Efforts*, GAO-09-334, February 26, 2009, http://www.gao.gov.

[12] Department of Homeland Security, *National Response Framework*, Washington, DC, January 2008, http://www.fema.gov/emergency/nrf/. See also CRS Report RL34758, *The National Response Framework: Overview and Possible Issues for Congress*, by Bruce R. Lindsay.

[13] For more information, see "Unclear Federal Leadership for Certain Response Functions," in CRS Report RL33579, *The Public Health and Medical Response to Disasters: Federal Authority and Funding*, by Sarah A. Lister.

[14] Department of Homeland Security, "Secretary Napolitano Issues Action Directives on First Responder Health Surge Capacity and Hurricane Katrina," press release, January 28, 2009, http://www.dhs.gov/ynews/releases.

[15] CRS Report RL33589, *The Pandemic and All-Hazards Preparedness Act (P.L. 109-417): Provisions and Changes to Preexisting Law*, by Sarah A. Lister and Frank Gottron.

[16] President George W. Bush, *Homeland Security Presidential Directive 21, Public Health and Medical Preparedness*, Washington, DC, October 18, 2007.

[17] General Services Administration, Federal Procurement Data System, contract transaction #1 8599705, September 30, 2008.

[18] CRS Report RL33579, *The Public Health and Medical Response to Disasters: Federal Authority and Funding*, by Sarah A. Lister. See, also, HHS, "Department of Health and Human Services Secretarial Declaration of a Public Heath Emergency," http://www.hhs.gov/disasters/discussion/planners/section319declaration.html.

[19] CRS Report RL34724, *Would an Influenza Pandemic Qualify as a Major Disaster Under the Stafford Act?*, by Edward C. Liu.

[20] CRS Report RL33589, *The Pandemic and All-Hazards Preparedness Act (P.L. 109-417): Provisions and Changes to Preexisting Law*, by Sarah A. Lister and Frank Gottron.

[21] See http://emergency.cdc.gov/cotper/coopagreement/.

[22] See http://www.hhs.gov/aspr/opeo/hpp/index.html.

[23] See, for example, Christopher D. Nelson, Ellen Burke Beckjord, and David J. Dausey, et al., "How Can We Strengthen the Evidence Base in Public Health Preparedness?," *Disaster Medicine and Public Health Preparedness*, vol. 2, no. 4 (December 2008), pp. 247-250; and

Nicole Lurie, Jeffrey Wasserman, and Christopher D. Nelson, "Public Health Preparedness: Evolution Or Revolution?," *Health Affairs*, vol. 25, no. 4 (July/August 2006), pp. 935-945.

[24] See Association of State and Territorial Health Officials, *States of Preparedness: Health Agency Progress, Second Edition*, Washington, DC, September 2008, http://www.astho.org/pubs/ StatesofPreparedness 2008fin.pdf; and U.S. Government Accountability Office, *Public Health and Hospital Emergency Preparedness Programs: Evolution of Performance Measurement Systems to Measure Progress*, GAO-07-485R, March 23, 2007, http://www.gao.gov.

[25] BARDA is in the Office of HHS/ASPR and is discussed in a subsequent section of this chapter, "Project BioShield".

[26] Subsequent to the passage of ARRA, Congress passed and the President signed P.L. 111-8, the Omnibus Appropriations Act, 2009, which provided funding for BARDA and pandemic flu, partly through transfers from an earlier FY2004 appropriation to the Department of Homeland Security for Project BioShield.

[27] For more information, see CRS Report R401 81, *Selected Health Funding in the American Recovery and Reinvestment Act of 2009*, coordinated by C. Stephen Redhead.

[28] See, for example, Eileen Salinsky, *Strong as the Weakest Link: Medical Response to a Catastrophic Event*, National Health Policy Forum, Background Paper No. 65, Washington, DC, August 8, 2008, http://www.nhpf.org/library/ details. cfm/2640; U.S. Government Accountability Office, *Emergency Preparedness: States Are Planning for Medical Surge, but Could Benefit from Shared Guidance for Allocating Scarce Medical Resources*, GAO-08-668, June 13, 2008, http://www.gao.gov; and Amy H. Kaji, Kristi L. Koenig, and Roger J. Lewis, "Current Hospital Disaster Preparedness," *JAMA*, vol. 298 (November 14, 2007), pp. 2188-2190.

[29] CRS Report RL33589, *The Pandemic and All-Hazards Preparedness Act (P.L. 109-417): Provisions and Changes to Preexisting Law*, by Sarah A. Lister and Frank Gottron.

[30] HHS: "HHS Supports Medical Evacuations in Preparation for Hurricane Gustav," press release, August 31, 2008; and "HHS Provides State Assistance in Preparing for Hurricane Ike, Recovering from Hurricane Gustav," press release, September 11, 2008, http://www.hhs.gov/news.

[31] See HHS, "Federal Public Health and Medical Assistance," http://www.hhs.gov/disasters/discussion/planners/medicalassistance.html.

[32] CRS Report RL33579, *The Public Health and Medical Response to Disasters: Federal Authority and Funding*, by Sarah A. Lister.

[33] CRS Report RL33738, *Gulf Coast Hurricanes: Addressing Survivors' Mental Health and Substance Abuse Treatment Needs*, by Ramya Sundararaman, Sarah A. Lister, and Erin D. Williams.

[34] See, for example, CRS Report RL32546, *Title VII Health Professions Education and Training: Issues in Reauthorization*, by Bernice Reyes-Akinbileje; and CRS Report RL32805, *Nursing Workforce Programs in Title VIII of the Public Health Service Act*, by Bernice Reyes-Akinbileje.

[35] CRS Report R40176, *Emergency Response: Civil Liability of Volunteer Health Professionals*, by Vivian S. Chu.

[36] CRS Report RL33589, *The Pandemic and All-Hazards Preparedness Act (P.L. 109-417): Provisions and Changes to Preexisting Law*, by Sarah A. Lister and Frank Gottron.

[37] HHS, *National Disaster Medical System*, http://www.hhs.gov/aspr/opeo/ndms/index.html.

[38] HHS, *About the Medical Reserve Corps*, http://www.medicalreservecorps.gov/About.

[39] U.S. Government Accountability Office, *Disaster Preparedness: Better Planning Would Improve OSHA 's Efforts to Protect Workers' Safety and Health in Disasters*, GAO-07-193, March 28, 2007, http:// www. gao. gov.

[40] Katherine Torres, "DHS Denies OSHA Power to Invoke Emergency Response Plan, Official Says," *Occupational Hazards*, vol. 70 (March 1, 2008); and "Despite Lawmakers' Concerns, OSHA's Role in NRF Remains Unchanged," *Inside OSHA*, February 4, 2008.

[41] NRF, Worker Safety and Health Support Annex, http://www.fema.gov/emergency/nrf/.

[42] For more information, see "Federal Assistance for Disaster-Related Health Care Costs," in CRS Report RL33579, *The Public Health and Medical Response to Disasters: Federal Authority and Funding*, by Sarah A. Lister; and CRS Report RL33927, *Selected Federal Compensation Programs for Physical Injury or Death*, Sarah A. Lister and C. Stephen Redhead, Coordinators.

[43] See HHS, "Emergency Awards for Healthcare Under Section 319 of the PHS Act Grants for Immediate Response," 67 *Federal Register* 15206-15208, March 29, 2002, the second of two notices of availability of funds. HHS invoked the public health emergency authority in Section 319 of the Public Health Service Act to support its action.

[44] For more information, see "World Trade Center Medical Monitoring and Treatment Program," in CRS Report RL33927, *Selected Federal Compensation Programs for Physical Injury or Death*, coordinated by Sarah A. Lister.

[45] U.S. Government Accountability Office, *Hurricane Katrina: Allocation and Use of $2 Billion for Medicaid and Other Health Care Needs*, GAO-07-67, February 28, 2007, http://www.gao.gov.

[46] For more information, see "World Trade Center Medical Monitoring and Treatment Program," in CRS Report RL33927, *Selected Federal Compensation Programs for Physical Injury or Death*, Sarah A. Lister and C. Stephen Redhead, Coordinators.

[47] The Security and Accountability For Every (SAFE) Port Act, P.L. 109-347, § 709, 120 Stat. 1947, Oct. 13, 2006.

[48] U.S. Government Accountability Office, *HHS Needs to Develop a Plan That Incorporates Lessons from the Responder Health Programs*, GAO-08-610, May 30, 2008, http://www.gao.gov.

[49] For more information, see "Unclear Federal Leadership for Certain Response Functions," in CRS Report RL33579, *The Public Health and Medical Response to Disasters: Federal Authority and Funding*, by Sarah A. Lister.

[50] U.S. Government Accountability Office, *September 11: HHS Needs to Develop a Plan That Incorporates Lessons from the Responder Health Programs*, GAO-08-610, May 30, 2008, http://www.gao.gov.

[51] Shortly before the 2005 hurricanes, the National Council on Disability issued a major report on emergency preparedness and individuals with disabilities. National Council on Disability, *Saving Lives: Including People with Disabilities in Emergency Planning*, Washington, DC, April 15, 2005, http://www.ncd.gov/ newsroom/ publications/ 2005/pdf/saving_lives.pdf.

[52] CRS Report RS22254, *The Americans with Disabilities Act and Emergency Preparedness and Response*, by Nancy Lee Jones.

[53] P.L. 110-161, the FY2008 Consolidated Appropriations Act, Division G, Title V, 121 Stat. 2213-2217; and HHS Administration for Children and Families, "Notification of the Establishment of the National Commission on Children and Disasters," 73 *Federal Register* 51489-51490, September 3, 2008. See also, the section "Children and Disasters" in CRS Report RL34758, *The National Response Framework: Overview and Possible Issues for Congress*, by Bruce R. Lindsay.

[54] U.S. Government Accountability Office, *National Disaster Response: FEMA Should Take Action to Improve Capacity and Coordination between Government and Voluntary Sectors*, GAO-08-369, February 27, 2008, http://www.gao.gov.

[55] CRS Report RS22576, *Pandemic Influenza: Appropriations for Public Health Preparedness and Response*, by Sarah A. Lister; and CRS Report RL33 145, *Pandemic Influenza: Domestic Preparedness Efforts*, by Sarah A. Lister.

[56] For more information, see HHS Pandemic Planning Updates I through VI, March 2006 through January 2009, http://www.pandemicflu.gov/plan/federal/index.html.

[57] Congressional Budget Office, *U.S. Policy Regarding Pandemic-Influenza Vaccines*, Washington, DC, September 2008, http://www.cbo.gov/doc.cfm?index=9573.

[58] U.S. Government Accountability Office, *Influenza Pandemic: Sustaining Focus on the Nation's Planning and Preparedness Efforts*, GAO-09-334, February 26, 2009, http://www.gao.gov.

[59] See HHS, *Assessment of States' Operating Plans to Combat Pandemic Influenza*, HHS Report to the Homeland Security Council, Washington, DC, January 2009, http://www.pandemicflu.gov/plan/states/index.html; and CRS Report RL34 190, *Pandemic Influenza: An Analysis of State Preparedness and Response Plans*, by Sarah A. Lister and Holly Stockdale.

[60] CRS Report RL34724, *Would an Influenza Pandemic Qualify as a Major Disaster Under the Stafford Act?*, by Edward C. Liu.

[61] CRS Report RL33201, *Federal and State Quarantine and Isolation Authority*, by Kathleen S. Swendiman and Jennifer K. Elsea; CRS Report RS22219, *The Americans with Disabilities Act (ADA) Coverage of Contagious Diseases*, by Nancy Lee Jones; and CRS Report RS21414, *Mandatory Vaccinations: Precedent and Current Laws*, by Kathleen S. Swendiman.

[62] CRS Report RL33609, *Quarantine and Isolation: Selected Legal Issues Relating to Employment*, by Nancy Lee Jones and Jon O. Shimabukuro.

[63] CRS Report RL34 144, *Extensively Drug-Resistant Tuberculosis (XDR-TB): Emerging Public Health Threats and Quarantine and Isolation*, by Kathleen S. Swendiman and Nancy Lee Jones.

[64] CRS Report RL3338 1, *The Americans with Disabilities Act (ADA): Allocation of Scarce Medical Resources During a Pandemic*, by Nancy Lee Jones.

[65] Commission on the Prevention of Weapons of Mass Destruction Proliferation and Terrorism, *World At Risk: The Report of the Commission on the Prevention of Weapons of Mass Destruction Proliferation and Terrorism*, New York, NY, December 2008, pp. 27-32, http://www.preventwmd.gov/home/.

[66] CRS Report R40418, *Oversight of High-Containment Biological Laboratories: Issues for Congress*, by Frank Gottron and Dana A. Shea.

[67] Laboratory oversight provisions are found in Title II of these bills. Provisions to reauthorize the Select Agent programs, discussed in the next section of this chapter, are found in Title I of these bills.

[68] 42 U.S.C. § 262a and 7 U.S.C. § 8401. See CDC Select Agent Program, http://www.cdc.gov/od/sap/, and APHIS Agricultural Select Agent Program, http://www.aphis.usda.gov/programs/ag_selectagent/.

[69] Federal Bureau of Investigation, "Anthrax Investigation: Closing a Chapter," August 6, 2008, http://www.fbi.gov/page2/august08/amerithrax080608a.html.

[70] Commission on the Prevention of Weapons of Mass Destruction Proliferation and Terrorism, *World At Risk: The Report of the Commission on the Prevention of Weapons of Mass Destruction Proliferation and Terrorism*, New York, NY, December 2008, pp. 27-32, http://www.preventwmd.gov/home/.

[71] U.S. Congress, Senate Committee on Homeland Security and Governmental Affairs, *Prevention of Weapons of Mass Destruction Proliferation and Terrorism*, 1 10th Cong., 2nd sess., December 11, 2008. See also Matthew M. Johnson, "Lieberman to Seek Tougher Regulations for Biological Research Labs," *CQ Homeland Security*, December 11, 2008.

[72] See, for example, testimony of the American Society for Microbiology, U.S. Congress, House Committee on Energy and Commerce, Subcommittee on Oversight and Investigations, hearing on *Creating the Department of Homeland Security: Consideration of the Administration's Proposal*, 107th Cong., 2nd sess., June 25, 2002.

[73] CRS Report RL33907, *Project BioShield: Appropriations, Acquisitions, and Policy Implementation Issues for Congress*, by Frank Gottron.

[74] In July, 2007, HHS published a draft plan. It has not been finalized. See HHS, Biomedical Advanced Research and Development Authority (BARDA), *Draft BARDA Strategic Plan*

for Medical Countermeasure Research, Development, and Procurement, Washington, DC, July 5, 2007, http://www.hhs.gov/ aspr/barda/ documents/ draftbardaplan.pdf.

[75] See, for example, U.S. Government Accountability Office, *Project Bioshield: Actions Needed to Avoid Repeating Past Mistakes*, GAO-08-208T, October 23, 2007, http://www.gao.gov.

[76] CRS Report RL32917, *Bioterrorism Countermeasure Development: Issues in Patents and Homeland Security*, by Wendy H. Schacht and John R. Thomas; and CRS Report RL33 159, *Influenza Antiviral Drugs and Patent Law Issues*, by Brian T. Yeh.

[77] CRS Report RS22327, *Pandemic Flu and Medical Biodefense Countermeasure Liability Limitation*, by Henry Cohen and Vanessa K. Burrows.

[78] Office of the Secretary, Department of Health and Human Services, 73 *Federal Register* 58239, October 6, 2008; and 73 *Federal Register* 61861-61873, October 17, 2008.

[79] An inventory of expired and expiring authorities, organized by congressional committees of jurisdiction, is provided in Congressional Budget Office, *Unauthorized Appropriations and Expiring Authorizations*, Washington, DC, January 2009, http://www.cbo.gov/doc.cfm?index=9960.

[80] CRS Report RL32546, *Title VII Health Professions Education and Training: Issues in Reauthorization*, by Bernice Reyes-Akinbileje.

[81] Public Health Service Act § 3 19F-2; 42 U.S.C. § 247d-6b. See CRS Report RL33589, *The Pandemic and All- Hazards Preparedness Act (P.L. 109-417): Provisions and Changes to Preexisting Law*, by Sarah A. Lister and Frank Gottron, for amendment to the program by the PAHPA.

In: Issues in Providing Emergency Medical Care ISBN: 978-1-61761-595-5
Editor: Mary E. Mathers

Chapter 5

AMBULANCE PROVIDERS: COSTS AND EXPECTED MEDICARE MARGINS VARY GREATLY

United States Government Accountability Office

WHY GAO DID THIS STUDY

In 2002, Medicare implemented a national fee schedule designed to standardize payments for ambulance services. The Medicare Prescription Drug, Improvement and Modernization Act of 2003 (MMA) required GAO to study ambulance service costs. GAO examined providers' costs of ground ambulance transports in 2004 and factors that contributed to cost differences; average Medicare ambulance payments expected under the national fee schedule in 2010 and how those payments will relate to providers' costs per transport; and changes that occurred in Medicare beneficiaries' use of ambulance transports from 2001 to 2004. GAO estimated costs of ambulance transports based on a nationally representative survey of 215 ambulance providers that did not share costs with nonambulance services. Providers that shared costs with other institutions or services and could not report their costs for ambulance services separately, such as fire departments, were excluded because their reported costs appeared unreliable. GAO used its survey, Medicare claims, and other data for its analyses.

What GAO Recommends

GAO recommends that the Administrator of CMS monitor utilization of ambulance transports to ensure that Medicare payments are adequate to provide for beneficiary access to ambulance services, particularly in super-rural areas. CMS agreed with GAO's recommendation.

What GAO Found

Costs of ground ambulance services were highly variable across providers that did not share costs with nonambulance services in 2004, reflecting differences in certain provider and community characteristics. Costs per transport among these providers varied from $99 per transport to $1,218. Providers without shared costs that had higher costs per transport typically had fewer transports per year, a greater percentage of transports in which more than a basic medical intervention occurred, more transports in super-rural areas (rural counties with lowest population density), lower productivity—measured as number of transports furnished per staffed hour, and a greater percentage of revenues from local tax support.

Average payments under the national fee schedule in 2010 are expected to be higher than historical payments, but providers' Medicare margins will vary greatly. GAO could not assess whether, on average, providers without shared costs would break even, lose, or profit under the national fee schedule, because the average Medicare margin for providers without shared costs was estimated to fall from negative 14 percent to positive 2 percent. However, GAO estimated that approximately 39 to 56 percent of providers without shared costs would have average Medicare payments above their average cost per transport under the national fee schedule in 2010.

From 2001 to 2004, utilization of ambulance transports per beneficiary increased 16 percent overall. However, use declined by 8 percent in super-rural areas.

Declining utilization coupled with potentially negative Medicare margins in super-rural areas, which could be exacerbated when the MMA temporary payment provisions expire, raise questions as to whether Medicare payments will be adequate to support beneficiary access in super-rural areas.

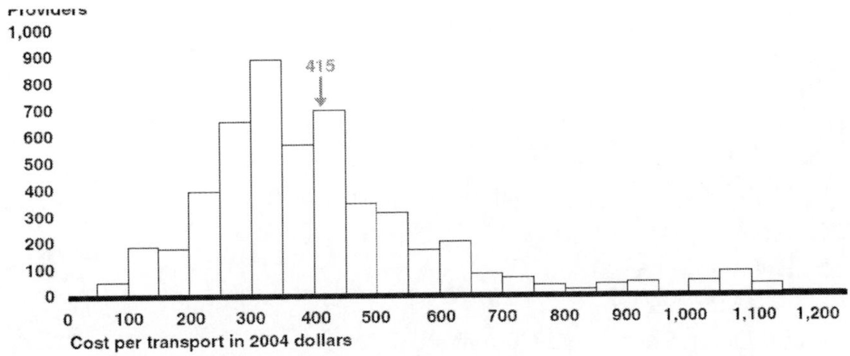

Source: 2005 GAO Survey of Ambulance Services.

Note: Based on a sample of 215 providers, weighted to represent more than 5,200 providers in the United States that did not share costs with nonambulance services.

Distribution of Cost per Transport for Providers without Shared Costs, 2004

ABBREVIATIONS

ALS	advanced life support
BLS	basic life support
CF	conversion factor
CMS	Centers for Medicare & Medicaid Services
CPI-U	Consumer Price Index for All Urban Consumers
EMS	emergency medical services
EMT	emergency medical technician
GPCI	geographic practice cost index
MMA	Medicare Prescription Drug, Improvement and Modernization Act of 2003
MSA	metropolitan statistical area
NECMA	New England county metropolitan area
NFS	national fee schedule
RVU	relative value unit

May 23, 2007

The Honorable Max Baucus
Chairman

The Honorable Charles E. Grassley
Ranking Member
Committee on Finance
United States Senate

The Honorable John D. Dingell
Chairman
The Honorable Joe Barton
Ranking Member
Committee on Energy and Commerce
House of Representatives

The Honorable Charles B. Rangel
Chairman
The Honorable Jim McCrery
Ranking Member
Committee on Ways and Means
House of Representatives

In 2005, ambulance service providers completed more than 12.6 million ground transports for Medicare beneficiaries.[1] Medicare paid more than $4 billion for ground ambulance transports and is likely the largest single payer of ambulance services in the United States.

As part of a series of Medicare payment reforms in 1997, Congress required the Health Care Financing Administration, now the Centers for Medicare & Medicaid Services (CMS), to develop a national fee schedule for Medicare ambulance services, which was implemented in 2002.[2] Historically, CMS had used two methods to pay for ambulance services, which resulted in wide variations in payment for the same service among different types of ambulance service providers. In particular, CMS had used one method—reasonable costs[3]—to pay hospital-based providers. It used another method—reasonable charges[4]—to pay other, nonhospitalbased types of ambulance service providers. This meant that hospital- based and nonhospital-based providers were paid different amounts for the same ambulance services.

In 2002, CMS began phasing in a national fee schedule that established a single payment method for all ambulance services regardless of the type of provider.[5] This fee schedule standardized Medicare payments for ambulance services. In general, providers strive to keep their costs of delivering a service at or below the standard fee schedule rate for that service. Under the Medicare ambulance national fee schedule, providers that have costs of delivering ambulance services above the fee schedule payment lose the difference between the payment amount and their costs, while providers with costs below the fee schedule payment are able to keep the difference between the payment amount and their costs. In aggregate, these differences are known as Medicare margins and express whether the provider makes a profit or loss on its Medicare transports. Some providers rely heavily on Medicare revenues and adequate Medicare margins help ensure the continuing availability of beneficiaries' access to ambulance services.

CMS phased in the ambulance national fee schedule from April 2002 through December 2005. During this transition, the new fee schedule payments were blended with the previous reasonable-cost payments for hospital-based providers and reasonable-charge payments for nonhospital-based providers. In 2003, Congress passed the Medicare Prescription Drug, Improvement and Modernization Act (MMA), which introduced several temporary payment provisions, including a regional fee schedule that overlapped with the transition to the national fee schedule.[6] Beginning in July 2004, these temporary payment provisions were expected to add about $840 million to Medicare payments for ambulance services through December 2009, when the last of these provisions are set to expire.

The Medicare, Medicaid, and SCHIP Benefits Improvement and Protection Act of 2000[7] and the MMA required GAO to study ambulance service costs. As discussed with the congressional committees of jurisdiction, in this chapter we (1) examined the differences in providers' costs of ambulance transports in 2004 and the factors that contributed to these cost differences, (2) assessed how the ambulance national fee schedule in 2010 is expected to affect average ambulance payments and how those payments will relate to providers' costs per transport, (3) determined the effect of MMA temporary payment provisions on ambulance payments, and (4) described the change that occurred in Medicare beneficiaries' use of ambulance transports from 2001 to 2004.

To examine differences in costs of providing ambulance transports, we conducted a national survey of ambulance providers in 2005. In our survey, we requested information about providers' costs, revenues, transports, and organizational characteristics for their most recently completed fiscal year.[8] We selected a stratified,[9] random sample of 500 eligible providers that billed Medicare, and we received 321 completed questionnaires for a response rate of 64 percent. We used this nationally representative sample of 321 providers to describe the ambulance industry.[10] However, after excluding two cost outliers, our analysis was further limited to a subgroup of providers that (1) did not share costs with other institutions or services or (2) shared costs but reported costs of ambulance services separately from the costs of their other services. Our analysis and findings are nationally representative of this subgroup of ambulance providers, which we refer to as providers without shared costs.[11] We excluded 104 providers that shared costs of ambulance services with other institutions or nonambulance services and could not distinguish their costs for providing ambulance services from other costs, including but not limited to all fire departments. We excluded these providers because their reported costs appeared to be unreliable. The resulting sample size for our analysis was 215 providers without shared costs. Although our sample is nationally representative of an estimated 5,200 providers without shared costs, the small sample size along with the variability of responses reduces the precision of our estimates, increasing the range of the 95 percent confidence intervals we report. A 95 percent confidence interval is the range within which we expect the true population estimate to fall 95 percent of the time, and it is the range of the confidence interval that expresses the precision of our estimates.

To examine factors that contributed to differences in costs, we used our survey data and Medicare data supplemented by data from two other sources. The Oil Price Information Service was our source for the average annual retail price of fuel by zip code, and the United States Postal Service supplied building rents because it tracks its facility costs in each zip code. We used regression analysis to analyze the relationships between various provider and local area characteristics and cost per transport among providers without shared costs. We also compared Medicare claims data for all nonrespondents with those of respondent providers without shared costs and determined that our cost estimates were not biased by nonresponse. See appendix I for details regarding our survey, other data sources, data limitations, and the analytic methods we employed.

To assess the effect of the ambulance national fee schedule on payments, we used Medicare claims data to compute average payments for ambulance transports in 2001, before the implementation of the ambulance national fee schedule, and in 2004, 2 years after the phase-in of the fee schedule had begun. For Medicare payment analyses, payments were expressed in 2004 dollars to exclude the effects of inflation. We also compared average payments for urban, rural, and super-rural transports.[12] We used Medicare claims data and payment formulas as specified in federal regulations to simulate average payments under the national fee schedule in 2010, after all of the MMA provisions expire, but computed these payments in 2004 dollars, the year that best reflects the cost data collected in our survey. To compare the simulated Medicare payments under the national fee schedule for providers without shared costs with the costs per transport of those providers, we computed providers' Medicare margins—the percentage difference between average Medicare payments and providers' costs per transport.[13] All costs per transport and provider margins are based solely on our sample of providers without shared costs, and for this reason, these estimates are reported with their confidence intervals.

We also assessed the effect of the MMA temporary payment provisions on payments in 2004 using Medicare claims data by examining the change in payments from the first half of the year, before the MMA changes went into effect, with the second half of the year, when MMA payment provisions had their maximum effect. To assess the change in Medicare beneficiaries' use of ambulance transports from 2001 to 2004, we used Medicare claims and CMS enrollment data, which contain information about beneficiaries, to compute transports per 1,000 beneficiaries for both years.

We tested the internal consistency and reliability of our survey data and all non-Medicare data sources and determined that all data sources were adequate for our purposes. We conducted our work from July 2004 through April 2007 in accordance with generally accepted government auditing standards.

RESULTS IN BRIEF

Costs of ground ambulance transports were highly variable across providers without shared costs, reflecting differences in certain provider characteristics. Costs per transport for providers without shared costs averaged $415, but varied from $99 to $1,218 per transport—a range of more than $1,100. Contributing to the variability were differences in providers' volume and mix of transports; service area (urban, rural, or super-rural); productivity, which we defined as the number of transports per staffed hour; and the percentage of total revenue derived from local tax support. Providers without shared costs had higher costs per transport when they had fewer transports per year, a greater percentage of transports in which more than a basic medical assessment or intervention occurred, and more transports from super-rural areas than providers without shared costs that did not have these characteristics. In addition, providers without shared costs that had lower productivity and those receiving a greater percentage of revenues from local tax support had higher costs per transport than providers without shared costs that had higher productivity and less local tax support. Other provider and local area characteristics, such as type of provider, region as determined by census division, building rent, and price of fuel, did not significantly affect average costs per transport among providers without shared costs.

Average payments under the national fee schedule in 2010, after all of the MMA temporary payment provisions are set to expire, are expected to be higher than payments in 2001, but Medicare margins for providers without shared costs will vary greatly. In 2010, average ambulance national fee schedule payments are estimated to be 3 percent higher overall than payments in 2001, after adjusting for inflation and assuming that providers bill the maximum amounts allowed. Further, a greater percentage than the overall increase in payments will accrue to rural and super-rural transports, on average, while urban transports will receive a decrease in payments under the national fee schedule in 2010. We could not assess whether providers without shared costs will break even, lose, or profit, on average, under the ambulance national fee schedule after the MMA temporary payment provisions expire, because the 95 percent confidence interval for the average expected Medicare margin for providers without shared costs spanned from negative 14 percent to positive 2 percent when we took into account the number of respondents in our sample and the range of their reported costs. However, across all providers without shared costs, we estimated that 39 to 56 percent will have average Medicare payments above their average costs per transport under the ambulance national fee schedule in 2010.

The MMA's temporary payment provisions, which included base- and mileage-rate increases as well as the introduction of a regional fee schedule, resulted in raised average ambulance payments overall, particularly for super-rural transports, which we determined were typically more costly to provide. However, regional payment adjustments by census division under the MMA did not appear to be warranted on the basis of regional cost differences. The regional fee schedule increased payments substantially for some regions but not others. After controlling for various characteristics that affected the costs of providing ambulance transports, we did not discern any significant differences in average cost per transport across regions.

From 2001 to 2004, Medicare beneficiaries' use of ambulance transports increased overall, even in those regions that had a decrease in average payments after the MMA was implemented. However, beneficiaries' use in super-rural areas decreased by 8 percent over the same period. The decline in the use of super-rural ambulance transports did not appear to be related to any significant change in the population of Medicare beneficiaries residing in super-rural areas.

In light of the variability in ambulance providers' Medicare margins and the potential for negative margins to have an impact on beneficiary access, we recommend that the Administrator of CMS monitor utilization of ambulance transports to ensure that Medicare payments are adequate to provide for beneficiary access to ambulance services, particularly in super-rural areas. In its comments on a draft of this chapter, CMS stated that it agreed with our recommendation. External commenters generally agreed with our findings.

BACKGROUND

Ground ambulance services are provided by a wide range of organizations that differ in their organizational structure, types of services offered, staffing, and revenue sources. Local conditions—including whether providers are affiliated with other organizations; whether their service areas are predominately urban, rural, or super-rural; and the amount of community-dedicated revenues—contribute to this diversity.

In addition, communities have few, if any, tools to help them decide the optimal organizational structure, staffing, or amount of funding for ambulance services, given local conditions. Although there have been efforts to establish national performance or quality standards,[14] there is limited information about how to best evaluate the costs of providing ambulance services in a community. In recent years, industry associations and federal agencies have worked to develop a data system and mechanisms for measuring the performance of emergency medical services (EMS); however, these tools cannot yet be applied to measure performance and evaluate the efficiency of ambulance services.[15] The lack of data and performance standards makes it difficult to assess whether any given provider is delivering quality care or whether services are being provided efficiently.

Organizational structures differ in that some ambulance providers are affiliated with another institution, such as a hospital or fire department, and in that providers may or may not offer other types of services, such as hospital services, fire suppression, rescue, or wheelchair transportation. Providers affiliated with another institution or that offer other types of services may share resources and operational costs, such as building space, administrative support, or personnel, with these other entities and services. About two-fifths of the ambulance industry shared operational costs with other institutions or services in 2004.[16] Nine percent of the ambulance industry was affiliated with a hospital, while 37 percent was affiliated with a fire department and 21 percent was affiliated with another government agency. Other communities (33 percent of the ambulance industry in 2004) were served by freestanding, for-profit or not-for-profit provider organizations.

The types of services offered and the staff employed also vary among providers. Some providers perform only emergency transports, in response to a 911 or equivalent call, while other providers offer nonemergency transports, which are typically transfers from one facility to another and may be scheduled in advance. In 2004, 45 percent of the ambulance industry performed only emergency transports; 55 percent performed emergency and nonemergency transports. Some providers perform only basic life support (BLS)[17] transports because their staff are not certified to perform more intensive medical assessments and interventions, such as advanced life support (ALS)[18] and other more complex services. In 2004, 9 percent of the ambulance industry specialized in only ALS and more complex Medicare transports, such as those requiring one or more ALS services or respiratory care; 14 percent performed only BLS Medicare transports; and 86 percent provided a mix of BLS, ALS, and more complex Medicare transports.[19] Fire departments are more likely to be specialized in ALS and more complex services. According to the fire departments that responded to our survey, 70 percent of their Medicare transports, on average, required ALS or more complex services; for other providers ALS and more complex transport services constituted only 49 percent of their Medicare transports.

Ambulance providers use of a variety of staff to deliver services to their communities. First, providers and communities determine what proportion of their staff will be emergency medical technicians (EMT) trained to perform BLS services, and what proportion will be EMT- intermediates or paramedics, who have training to perform more intensive ALS interventions.[20] In 2004, 77 percent of providers that completed our survey reported having at least one staff member trained as a paramedic, nurse, or physician, but the remaining 23 percent of respondent providers relied on staff with less training than a paramedic. Other staffing choices include whether to employ career-oriented paid staff, rely on volunteers, or use a mix of paid and volunteer staff. Some providers choose to employ cross-trained staff.[21] In 2004, two-fifths of the ambulance industry relied substantially on volunteer staff.[22] In addition, providers and communities make different choices about whether to maintain backup vehicles and staff or to rely to a greater extent on nearby providers for backup assistance.

Providers' service areas can be urban, rural, super-rural, or a mix of areas. During 2004, CMS defined urban transports as those that originate within metropolitan statistical areas (MSA) and New England county metropolitan areas (NECMA), rural transports as those that originate in rural counties that are outside of MSAs and NECMAs,[23] and super-rural transports as those that originate in the bottom 25 percent of rural areas as defined by population density. About half of the ambulance providers served predominately urban areas, and the other half served predominately rural and super-rural areas.[24] However, three-fourths of all Medicare transports originated in urban areas. Therefore, rural and super- rural providers performed fewer transports on average than urban providers. In addition, rural and super-rural transports were longer than urban transports, on average, requiring more time and resources per transport. In 2004, urban Medicare transports averaged 7 miles, while rural Medicare transports averaged 13 miles and Medicare transports from super-rural areas averaged 20 miles.

Providers have several potential revenue sources depending on their communities and their choices about funding ambulance services. Revenue sources can include community tax support (such as revenue from local governments); charitable donations; state and federal grants; subscription programs;[25] and reimbursements from Medicare or Medicaid patients, and private health insurance companies. Not all providers receive revenues from all sources, and the mix and amount of revenues available may vary.[26] For example, 48 percent of the ambulance industry indicated that a state or local government approves the fees they may choose to charge. In communities that limit ambulance providers' fees, providers may bill Medicare (and other payers) less than the allowed amount and therefore do not receive the maximum Medicare payment allowed for their services. In 2004, Medicare payments for ambulance transports accounted for 31 percent of the providers' revenues, on average, while Medicare beneficiaries accounted for about 40 percent of their transports during that same year.[27] However, the percentage of Medicare revenues among providers ranged from less than 1 percent to 80 percent. Furthermore, different communities provide different levels of tax support to address specific issues, such as ensuring a minimum level of service in remote areas or being equipped with more sophisticated transport vehicles or having more highly trained staff.

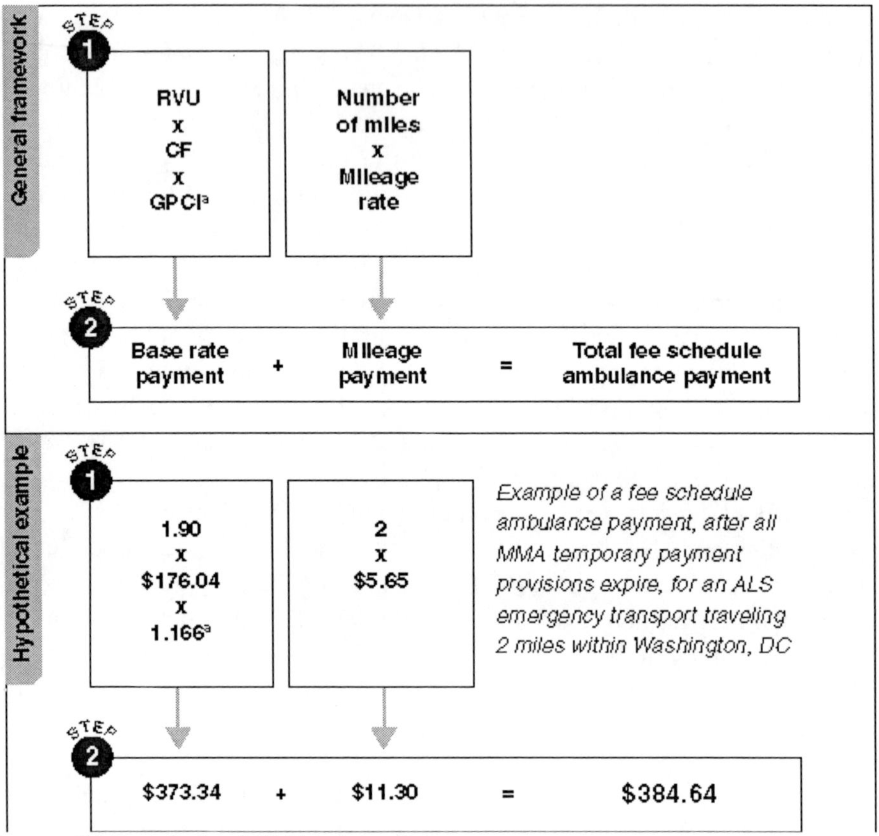

Source: GAO analysis of CMS information.

Note: Payments are expressed in 2004 dollars.

[a] The GPCI is applied to only 70 percent of the unadjusted base rate payment, which is the product of the RVU and the CF. For example, the base rate payment equals 1.90 x $176.04 x [0.30 + (0.70 x 1.166)]. The RVU, CF, GPCI, and mileage rate are based on 2004 values.

Figure 1. Medicare Ambulance Payment Formula under the National Fee Schedule

Medicare Ambulance National Fee Schedule

The ambulance national fee schedule was part of a series of payment reforms to make Medicare a more equitable and prudent purchaser of health care services. Phased in from April 2002 through December 2005, the national fee schedule standardized payment rates and reduced wide variations in payments for the same service.

Medicare ambulance payments under the fee schedule have two components: a base-rate payment and a mileage payment.[28] The base-rate component of ambulance payments under the fee schedule consists of the relative value unit (RVU), the conversion factor (CF), and a geographic adjustment factor. Ambulance RVUs account for the relative resources needed to provide services during an ambulance transport.[29] The ambulance CF converts the RVU into a payment expressed in dollars and is set by CMS annually. Ambulance base-rate payments are also adjusted by a geographic practice cost index (GPCI), which is intended to account for regional differences in the cost of providing ambulance services.[30] The mileage component consists of the number of miles traveled during an ambulance transport multiplied by the applicable mileage rate. (See figure 1 for an example of the payment formula.[31])

The ambulance national fee schedule was phased in from April 2002 through December 2005 by blending new fee schedule payments with historical payments. During this transition, the national fee schedule portion constituted a greater share of the total blended ambulance payment each year until January 2006, when the historical payment portion of the blend was discontinued. For example, in the latter part of 2002, total ambulance payments were a blend of 20 percent under the national fee schedule and 80 percent under the historical payment system. In 2004, the blend was 60 percent national fee schedule and 40 percent historical payment system. (See figure 2 for further details on the blending of historic payments and national fee schedule payments.)

MMA Temporary Payment Provisions

The MMA introduced several temporary ambulance payment provisions that were implemented in 2004, the last of which expires at the end of 2009. CMS estimates that these payment adjustments will add $840 million to Medicare ambulance services over the 5 years they are in effect. The MMA provisions increased payment rates for urban and rural transports and for transports 51 miles or greater. The MMA also provided a significant base rate increase for transports originating in super-rural areas and provided for a new regional fee schedule based on the nine census divisions.[32]

The regional fee schedule was designed to ease the transition from the historical payment system to the national fee schedule. The introduction of the regional fee schedule overlapped with the phase-in of the national fee schedule. The regional fee schedule gave temporarily higher ambulance payments than what would generally be paid under the national fee schedule to ambulance providers in census divisions that had historically higher payments. If the regional base-rate payment was determined to be greater than the national base-rate payment for a particular region, then the region received the more advantageous blend of the regional fee schedule base-rate payment and the national fee schedule base-rate payment. For example, in the second half of 2004 under the regional fee schedule, affected regions received a blend of 80 percent of their regional fee schedule base-rate payment and 20 percent of the national fee schedule base payment rate. This base-rate payment was then further blended with historical payments as a part of the gradual phase-in of the ambulance national fee schedule.[33] The regional fee schedule component of the base rate blend was reduced each year from 2005 through 2007, and expires at the end of 2009. (See figure 2 for further details on the blending of historical, national fee schedule, and regional fee schedule payments.)

Table 1. Summary of MMA Temporary Payment Provisions, Implemented July 1, 2004

Payment provision	Expiration date
The regional fee schedule	December 31, 2009
An increase in the base rate for super-rural transports[a]	December 31, 2009
A 25 percent increase in the urban and rural mileage rate for every ambulance mile exceeding 50	December 31, 2008
A 1 percent and 2 percent increase for urban and rural transports and mileage, respectively	December 31, 2006

Source: 42 U.S.C. § 1395m(l)(10)-(13).

[a] CMS determined that this increase would be approximately 23 percent. 69 *Fed. Reg.* 40288 (July 1, 2004).

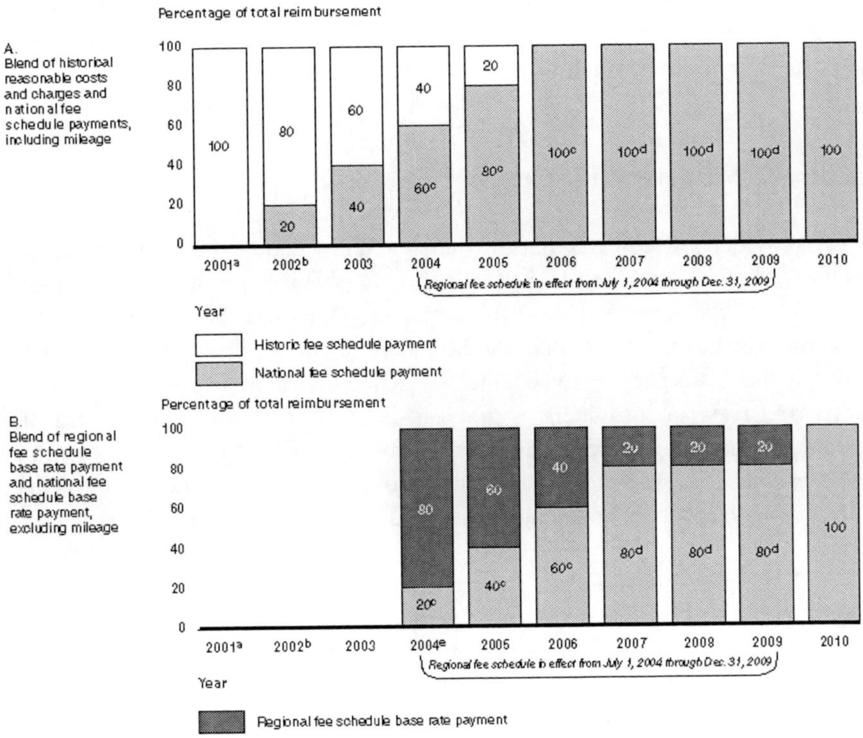

Source: GAO analysis of CMS information.

Note: All years refer to calendar years unless otherwise specified.

Figure 2. National Fee Schedule and Regional Fee Schedule

[a] January 1, 2001 through March 31, 2002.

[b] April 1, 2002 through December 31, 2002.

[c] The national fee schedule payment portion includes MMA increases of 1 percent and 2 percent for urban and rural transports, respectively, and an approximate 23 percent base rate increase for super- rural transports.

[d] The national fee schedule payment portion includes an MMA base rate increase of approximately 23 percent for super-rural transports only.

[e] July 1, 2004 through December 31, 2004.

In addition to providing for a regional fee schedule, the MMA temporarily required higher payment rates for super-rural transports. As a result, base rate payments for transports originating in super-rural areas increased about 23 percent. The MMA also provided for a 25 percent increase in the mileage rate for every ambulance mile traveled exceeding 50. Finally, the MMA required an increase in payment rates for mileage and transports originating in urban and rural areas by 1 percent and 2 percent, respectively. (See table 1 for MMA temporary payment provisions and their expiration dates.)

Medicare Margins and Costs

A provider's Medicare margin under a fee schedule generally depends on whether the provider's costs of delivering a service are below its Medicare payments for the service. Under the ambulance national fee schedule, providers with costs per transport less than the Medicare payment for that transport are able to retain the difference between the fee schedule payment and their costs per transport. Likewise, providers with costs per transport above the national fee schedule payment will lose the difference between the Medicare payment and their costs per transport. Therefore, ambulance providers that can control their costs per transport may have an advantage over those that cannot control their costs per transport.

A 2003 GAO study found that transport costs are likely to be higher in less densely populated rural areas because rural providers furnish fewer transports and because fewer transports were linked to higher costs per transport.[34] As a result, we recommended that CMS adjust payments for transports in rural counties with particularly low population density to help ensure Medicare beneficiaries' access to ambulance services in those areas. Subsequently, the MMA increased payments for super-rural transports from July 1, 2004, through December 31, 2009. The report also found that the majority of ambulance providers' costs were related to readiness—the availability of ambulance and crew for immediate emergency response—and were fixed costs. Fixed costs, such as staff on call, vehicles, building space, and administration, generally do not increase as the number of transports increases. Fuel costs and supplies are not fixed costs because they increase with the number of transports.

Costs per Transport Were Highly Variable, Reflecting Differences in Certain Provider Characteristics

Costs of ground ambulance transports were highly variable across providers without shared costs; an average ambulance transport ranged from a low of $99 to a high of $1,218 during 2004, the year for which we gathered data. The variability of costs per transport reflected differences in certain characteristics—volume and mix of transports; service areas (urban, rural, and super-rural); productivity, which we defined as transports per staffed hour; and amount of local tax support.[35] As expected, low volume, a greater percentage of ALS and more complex transports, and more transports from super-rural areas were key characteristics that helped explain why some providers without shared costs had higher costs per transport. Two other provider characteristics— productivity and amount of local tax support—were also associated with higher costs per transport for providers without shared costs. Other provider and local area characteristics—such as type of provider, region, building rent, and price of fuel—did not significantly affect average costs per transport among providers without shared costs.

Providers' Reported Costs per Transport Were Highly Variable

Providers' average costs for a ground ambulance transport varied from $99 to $1,218—a range of more than $1,100—across providers without shared costs in 2004. Figure 3 shows the wide variation in the reported costs per transport among providers without shared costs. Five percent of providers without shared costs had average costs per transport that were less than $152, while 5 percent of providers had average costs per transport more than $913. From our sample of providers without shared costs, we estimated the average cost per transport at $415, with a 95 percent confidence interval—the range within which we expect the population average cost per transport to fall 95 percent of the time—of $381 to $450.[36] This means that the actual average cost per transport across ambulance providers in the United States without shared costs was from $381 to $450 in 2004.

When we categorized providers without shared costs by service area and compared the average costs per transport across the groups, average cost per transport among super-rural providers was statistically significantly different from that of urban providers, but rural providers' average cost per transport was not statistically significantly different from that of urban providers. The average cost per transport for super-rural providers without shared costs was $538,[37] statistically significantly different from the $370 average cost per transport for urban providers without shared costs. The 95 percent confidence interval for average costs per transport among super-rural providers without shared costs ranged from $448 to $628 and among urban providers without shared costs ranged from $326 to $414. The average cost per transport among rural providers without shared costs was $409 within a confidence interval spanning $354 to $465, an interval that overlapped with the average costs per transport estimates for both urban and super-rural providers without shared costs.

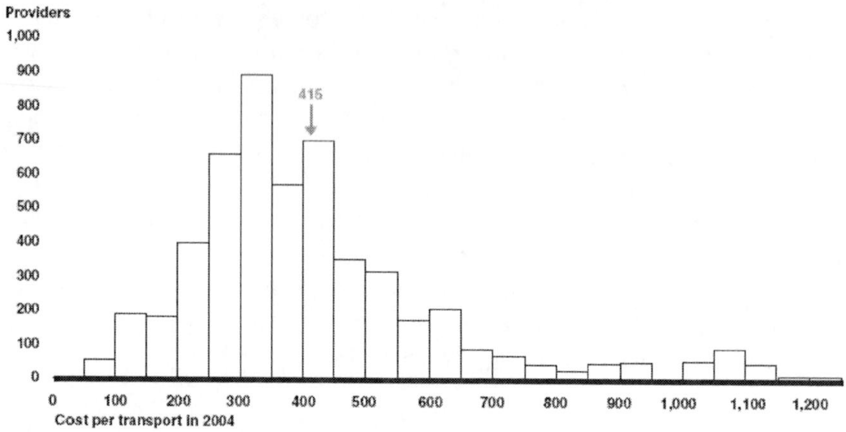

Source: 2005 GAO Survey of Ambulance Services.

Note: Based on a sample of 215 providers, weighted to represent more than 5,200 providers in the United States that did not share costs with nonambulance services.

Figure 3. Distribution of Cost per Transport for Providers without Shared Costs in 2004

Certain Provider Characteristics Contributed to Differences in Costs per Transport

The variability of costs per transport among providers without shared costs reflected differences in certain provider characteristics. The provider characteristics that contributed to significant differences in costs per transport were volume, mix of transports, service area, productivity, and amount of local tax support.[38] (See table 2 and app. I for a full description of our methods.)

Providers without shared costs that had lower transport volumes generally had higher average costs than providers without shared costs with higher transport volumes. Our analysis affirms the finding of our prior work, that volume of transports was the main characteristic affecting providers' costs per transport.[39] Because most ambulance costs are fixed, and therefore do not increase significantly when a provider completes more transports, it is expected that as the number of transports provided increases, associated costs per transport will be lower. In 2004, the volume of transports completed by a provider without shared costs ranged from 21 to more than 50,000. Estimated average cost per transport is reduced, from $464 for providers without shared costs completing 2,000 or fewer transports a year to $327 for those completing from 3,001 to 4,000 transports. Although estimated average cost per transport is slightly higher for 4,001 to 5,000 transports, rising to $330, and again above 6,000 transports, rising to $330, every other volume category of provider without shared costs had lower estimated average costs per transport than the lowest volume group of 2,000 transports or less.

Table 2. Estimated Average Cost per Transport for Provider Characteristics That Affect Costs

	Assigned values	Estimated average cost per transport[a]
Volume of transports	2,000 or less	$464
	2,001 – 3,000	388
	3,001 – 4,000	327
	4,001 – 5,000	330
	5,001 – 6,000	276
	6,001 or more	330
Mix of transports	Only BLS	360
	ALS or more intensive services	476
Service area	Urban only	358
	Rural only	420[b]
	Super-rural only	545
Productivity—transports per staffed hour	1 transport per 8 hours (0.12)	437
	5 transports per 8 hours (0.64)	386
Local tax support	No tax support	392
	Local tax support as 81% of revenues	632

Sources: GAO analysis of 2005 GAO Survey of Ambulance Services and 2004 Medicare claims.

[a] The estimated average cost per transport is for providers without shared costs. It was created by assigning a value to the provider characteristic of interest for all cases and using the national average value for the other characteristics. See app. I. for detailed information about our methods.

[b] The estimated cost of a rural transport was not significantly different from the estimated cost of an urban transport.

Also, as expected, we observed that average costs per transport were higher for providers without shared costs that also had a greater percentage of

ALS and more complex transports (compared with BLS transports) and those with a greater percentage of super-rural transports (compared with urban transports)—two characteristics incorporated into the national fee schedule to account for the additional costliness associated with more intensive services and isolated service areas. ALS and more complex transports completed by providers without shared costs ranged from 0 to 100 percent of transports provided. We estimated that providers without shared costs specializing in ALS and more complex transport services had average costs of $476, which was 32 percent higher than providers without shared costs specializing in BLS transport services. We estimated that the average cost of a super-rural transport was $545,[40] while the average cost of an urban transport was $358. Rural transports were not significantly higher cost than urban transports.

Two other provider characteristics—productivity and amount of local tax support—were also associated with higher average costs per transport. Costs were higher when providers without shared costs had lower productivity or a lower ratio of transports per staffed hour. The average level of productivity for providers without shared costs was 0.12, or about one transport per 8 staffed hours, and had an estimated average cost per transport of $437. The second highest level of productivity for these providers was 0.64, or more than five transports per 8 staffed hours, and had an estimated average cost per transport of $386. The impact of productivity on average costs may be explained by the fixed costs incurred in maintaining readiness—having an ambulance and crew available to respond to emergency calls. Although providers may have discretion about staffing and the ability to make backup arrangements to substitute for additional staff, not all providers can increase productivity by increasing the number of transports they provide or reducing the number of staffed ambulance hours. For example, providers that operate in small or isolated communities with one ambulance on call may serve only their own community's needs and may not be able to expand their service area or increase their volume of ambulance transports.

Average costs were also higher for providers without shared costs that derived a larger percentage of their total revenues from local tax support. Among providers without shared costs, those with the largest percentage of revenues from local tax support (81 percent of revenues) had estimated average costs that were $240, or 61 percent, above those with no local tax support. Again, this effect was independent of volume and mix of transports, service area, cost of labor, use of volunteers, productivity, and other provider and local area characteristics. The relationship between greater local tax support and higher average costs may be explained as the income effect: if an organization has more money, it is able to and likely to spend more. Moreover, if costs increase without resulting in additional transports, the average cost per transport will increase.

Characteristics that did not significantly contribute to the variability of average costs per transport among providers without shared costs included type of provider; a provider's region, as measured by the nine census divisions that defined the regional fee schedule; building rent; and the price of fuel.

Average Payments under the National Fee Schedule Will Be Greater Than Average Historical Payments, but Providers' Expected Medicare Margins Will Vary Greatly

Average ambulance national fee schedule payments in 2010 are estimated to be 3 percent higher overall than payments in 2001, after adjusting for inflation and assuming that providers bill the maximum amounts allowed. However, the Medicare margins of providers without shared costs— whether they make a profit or a loss on Medicare transports—will vary under the national fee schedule. We cannot assess whether providers without shared costs will break even, lose, or profit on average under the ambulance national fee schedule in 2010 after all of the MMA temporary payment provisions have expired, because the 95 percent confidence interval surrounding the average Medicare margin spans from negative 14 percent to positive 2 percent. However, across all providers without shared costs, we estimate that 39 to 56 percent will have average Medicare payments above their average costs per transport under the ambulance national fee schedule even after all of the MMA provisions expire.

Average Payments under the National Fee Schedule Will Be Greater Than Average Historical Payments and Will Be Redistributed from Urban Transports to Rural and Super-Rural Transports

Compared with average historical payments in 2001, average payments under the national fee schedule in 2010 will be 3 percent higher, after adjusting for inflation and assuming providers will bill the maximum amount allowed under the national fee schedule. According to our analysis, urban transports will experience a decrease in payments, on average, while rural and super-rural transports will receive an increase that is greater than the overall increase. Average payments for rural and super-rural transports will increase 20 percent and 15 percent, respectively, while average payments for urban transports will decline 3 percent compared with average payments prior to the fee schedule. (See table 3.)

Expected Medicare Margins Will Vary Greatly

After all of the MMA temporary payment provisions expire, expected Medicare margins under the national fee schedule will vary greatly among providers without shared costs. When we compared expected payments under the national fee schedule in 2010 with providers' costs per transport, the resulting Medicare margins ranged from negative 194 percent for one provider to positive 76 percent for another provider. This wide difference is related to the great variability in reported costs among providers without shared costs.

Table 3. Payments Prior to and under the National Fee Schedule after MMA Provisions Expire

Transports	Payment prior to national fee schedule	Payments under national fee schedule	Percentage change
Urban	$309	$301	-3
Rural	303	363	20
Super-rural	379	437	15
National	309	319	3

Sources: GAO analysis of 2001 and 2004 Medicare claims.

Notes: All payments are in 2004 dollars. Payments under the national fee schedule assume that providers charge the maximum allowed amount.

Table 4. Expected Average Medicare Margins under the National Fee Schedule for Providers without Shared Costs in 2004 Dollars

Providers' predominate service area	Payment under national fee schedule	Average cost (95 percent confidence interval)	Providers' average Medicare margins in percentage (95 percent confidence interval)
Urban	$350	$370 (326 to 414)	-6 (-18 to 6)
Rural	408	409 (354 to 465)	-1 (-13 to 12)
Super-rural	471	538 (448 to 628)	-17 (-35 to 2)
All	394	415 (381 to 450)	-6(-14 to 2)

Sources: GAO analysis of 2005 GAO Survey of Ambulance Services and 2004 Medicare claims.

Notes: All payments and costs are in 2004 dollars. Payments under the national fee schedule assume that providers charge the maximum allowed amount. The range of the confidence interval is affected by the variability of costs per transport within the sample and the size of the sample. Providers' average Medicare margin is the average margin across all providers in the sample.

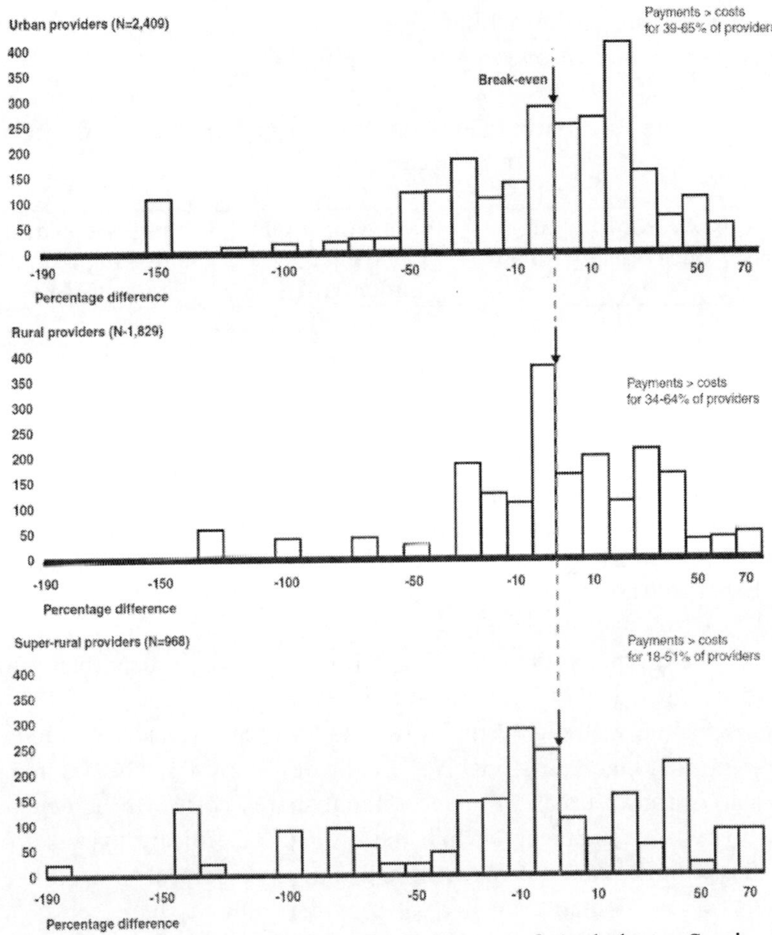

Sources: GAO analysis of 2005 GAO Survey of Ambulance Services and 2004 Medicare claims.

Notes: The range of the confidence interval is affected by the variability of costs per transport within the sample and the size of the sample. Percentages and confidence intervals are rounded.

Figure 4. Expected Medicare Margins for Urban, Rural, and Super-Rural Providers without Shared Costs

Among providers without shared costs, we estimated that the average Medicare margin, or the average percentage difference between these providers' Medicare payments and their costs, will be about negative 6 percent with a 95 percent confidence interval from negative 14 percent to positive 2 percent. (See table 4.) This span in the confidence interval means we cannot assess whether providers without shared costs would break even, lose, or profit, on average, under the national fee schedule in 2010 after all of the MMA temporary payment provisions have expired.

Table 5. Average Payments Prior to MMA Implementation and after Implementation

Transports	Average payment per transport prior to MMA	Average payment Per transport under MMA	Average percentage change in payment under MMA
Urban	$306	$322	5
Rural	358	370	3
Super-rural	442	497	12
National	322	338	5

Source: GAO analysis of 2004 Medicare claims.

Notes: The period prior to MMA implementation for which payments were computed was January 1, 2004 through June 30, 2004. The period after implementation of the MMA for which payments were computed was July 1, 2004 through December 31, 2004.

Similarly, we estimated that the average Medicare margin for urban, rural, and super-rural providers without shared costs will be negative under the national fee schedule, but each estimate will fall within a broader confidence interval range that includes positive Medicare margins. The estimated Medicare margin for an urban provider without shared costs will be negative 18 percent to positive 6 percent, while the estimated Medicare margin for a rural provider without shared costs will be negative 13 percent to positive 12 percent. We estimated that a super-rural provider without shared costs will have an estimated Medicare margin from negative 35 percent to positive 2 percent, making it more likely that the average Medicare margin for any given super-rural provider without shared costs would be negative rather than positive. However, given the confidence intervals surrounding the estimated average margin for each subset of providers without shared costs and the lack of statistical difference between them, we cannot conclude with certainty that any subset of providers would have significantly better or worse financial experience under Medicare's national fee schedule than another. Rather, we can conclude only that Medicare margins are likely to vary even among urban, rural, and super-rural providers without shared costs.

When we assessed the likely experiences of all providers without shared costs under the national fee schedule after all of the MMA temporary payment provisions expire, we estimated that 39 to 56 percent of them will have positive Medicare margins. Among urban and rural providers, 39 to 65 percent and 34 to 64 percent, respectively, will have positive Medicare margins, according to our estimations. Among super-rural providers, however, we estimate that 18 to 51 percent will have positive Medicare margins, while 49 to 82 percent would have zero or negative Medicare margins. (See figure 4.) The breadth of these confidence intervals reflects the variability of providers' costs in 2004 and expected financial experience under the national fee schedule after MMA temporary payment provisions expire.

MMA Provisions Resulted in Greater Average Payments for Higher-Cost Super-Rural Transports and Adjusted Payments Regionally Where No Significant Cost Differences Were Observed

The MMA temporary payment provisions, which were implemented by CMS in the second half of 2004, resulted in raised ambulance average payments overall, particularly for super-rural transports, which we found typically more costly to provide. Payment adjustments under the MMA's regional fee schedule were not justified on the basis of regional cost differences, as we did not find significant differences in average cost per transport across regions.

Payment Increases Were Targeted to Higher-Cost Super-Rural Transports

When we compared ambulance payments in the first half of 2004, prior to the implementation of the MMA provisions, with ambulance payments in the second half of 2004, after the temporary payment provisions were implemented and had their maximum effect, we found that payments, on average, increased by 5 percent overall. Super-rural transports received more substantial payment increases than urban or rural transports. (See table 5.) After MMA temporary payment provisions were implemented, average payments for urban and rural transports increased by 5 and 3 percent, respectively, while average payments for super-rural transports rose by 12 percent, compared with average payments before the MMA provisions were implemented. Increased payments for super-rural transports under the MMA were in keeping with our finding that super- rural transports were more costly than urban transports, independent of other characteristics that affected ambulance costs.

Regional Payment Adjustments Required by the MMA Were Not Justified on the Basis of Regional Cost Differences

Regional payment adjustments under the MMA were not warranted on the basis of regional cost differences. The MMA required a regional fee schedule, which resulted in ambulance payments for similar services that differed based on the region where they were provided. When comparing average regional payments before the implementation of MMA provisions to payments after implementation of the MMA, when the regional fee schedule had its greatest effect, we found that average payments increased substantially for some regions but not others. (See table 6.) However, we found no significant differences in costs by region, after controlling for differences in volume and mix of transports, cost of labor, service area, and other characteristics that may have affected costs. The regional fee schedule is due to expire on December 31, 2009.

Table 6. Percentage Changes in Average Payments prior to MMA Implementation and after Implementation, by Region

Region	Percentage change in average payments
Pacific	19
New England	12
Mountain	8
West South Central	7
West North Central	3
Middle Atlantic	3
South Atlantic	1
East North Central	1
East South Central	0

Source: GAO analysis of 2004 Medicare claims.

Notes: East South Central received a decrease in average payments of -0.04 percent, which rounds to 0 percent. The period prior to MMA implementation for which payments were computed was January 1, 2004 through June 30, 2004. The period after implementation of the MMA for which payments were computed was July 1, 2004 through December 31, 2004. See table 11 in app. I for a listing of the regions, or census divisions, and their corresponding states.

Table 7. Ambulance Transports per 1,000 Beneficiaries in Urban, Rural, and Super- Rural Areas

Area	Transports, 2001	Transports, 2004	Percentage change, 2001-2004
Urban	371	443	19
Rural	372	396	6
Super-rural	264	244	-8
Total	**364**	**420**	**16**

Sources: GAO analysis of 2001 and 2004 Medicare claims and CMS enrollment data.

MEDICARE BENEFICIARIES' USE OF AMBULANCE TRANSPORTS INCREASED FROM 2001 TO 2004, EXCEPT IN SUPER-RURAL AREAS

Nationally, the use of ambulance transports by Medicare beneficiaries increased by 16 percent, from 2001, the year before the transition to the national fee schedule began, to 2004, the year we studied. (See table 7.) Medicare beneficiaries' use of ambulance transports in urban areas experienced the greatest growth, 19 percent, while rural areas experienced a modest increase of 6 percent. However, Medicare transports per 1,000 beneficiaries in super-rural areas decreased by 8 percent. The decrease in Medicare beneficiaries' use of ambulance transports in super-rural areas was driven mostly by a decline in the volume of transports rather than any significant change in the number of beneficiaries or the demographic characteristics of beneficiaries residing in super-rural areas. For example, factors such as age, race, and gender remained stable in the super-rural Medicare population. Meanwhile, Medicare beneficiaries' use of ambulance transports increased in all regions from 2001 to 2004, including one region that had a decrease in average payments under the MMA compared with before the implementation of MMA payment provisions.

CONCLUSIONS

The diversity of the ambulance industry is reflected in its range of organizations, services offered, staffing, revenue sources, and costs per transport. We found that certain ambulance provider characteristics, such as volume, mix of transports, service area, productivity, and amount of local tax support, affected the cost per transport of providers without shared costs. For some providers and communities, these characteristics may be self-determined and may reflect those communities' preferences for readiness, quality standards, and ambulance services offered. For example, some communities may prefer to fund the greater costs of operating at a higher level of readiness or being equipped with more sophisticated transport vehicles and more highly trained staff. Other providers and communities have little or no control over the characteristics that affect providers' cost per transport. These communities, particularly more rural areas with low population density, may be constrained by local conditions, including their financial resources. Therefore, local conditions and community preferences may explain some of the predicted variability in the financial experience of providers without shared costs under the Medicare national fee schedule.

We are unable to discern whether providers without shared costs would be compensated appropriately under the national fee schedule for two reasons. First, when providers experience the national fee schedule payments in 2010 after all of the MMA temporary payment provisions expire, they may make changes to control or reduce their costs. The cost data we collected were from 2004 and may not reflect any changes providers may make to control or reduce their costs in response to the national fee schedule. Second, we did not assess if Medicare beneficiaries are receiving quality care that is delivered efficiently. There are no national performance standards to use as benchmarks for determining quality and efficiency of services or for assessing whether providers could increase productivity by increasing the number of transports they provide or by reducing the number of staffed ambulance hours. However, current efforts to develop a national data system and indicators for EMS systems may, in the future, yield useful tools for measuring efficiency and quality of ambulance services under the Medicare program.

Based on our survey of ambulance costs, we were able to estimate that some providers without shared costs would have positive Medicare margins under the national fee schedule after the MMA provisions expire, while others would have negative Medicare margins. Among super-rural providers, we estimated that 18 to 51 percent would have positive Medicare margins. However, 49 to 82 percent would have zero or negative Medicare margins. Ideally, Medicare payments should be adequate to ensure beneficiary access to services while using the program's resources judiciously. The decline in use of super-rural ground ambulance transports from 2001 to 2004, a time when payments for super-rural transports were increased, suggests that Medicare payment levels may not be linked to the decreased utilization of transports in super-rural areas. However declining utilization coupled with potentially negative Medicare margins in super- rural areas, which could be exacerbated when the MMA provisions expire, raise questions as to whether Medicare payments will be adequate to support beneficiary access in super-rural areas.

Recommendation for Executive Action

In light of the variability in ambulance providers' Medicare margins and the potential for negative margins to have an impact on beneficiary access, we recommend that the Administrator of CMS monitor utilization of ambulance transports to ensure that Medicare payments are adequate to provide for beneficiary access to ambulance services, particularly in super-rural areas.

Agency and External Comments and Our Evaluation

We provided a draft of this chapter to CMS and to five associations that represent the ambulance industry: the American Ambulance Association, the National Association of State EMS Officials, the National Ambulance Coalition, the National Volunteer Fire Council, and the International Association of Fire Chiefs. CMS's written comments are reprinted in appendix II.

CMS stated that, for the most part, the report reinforces its findings. CMS also stated that it agreed with our recommendation that the agency monitor utilization of ambulance transports to ensure that Medicare payments are adequate to provide for beneficiary access to ambulance services, particularly in super-rural areas. CMS noted that it would continue to monitor ambulance rates and would make adjustments should the original assumptions made during the development of the ambulance fee schedule need to be changed. In addition, CMS also highlighted its implementation of a refinement in the definition of rural areas that should enable rural areas within urban areas to receive the benefit of higher rural payments under the ambulance fee schedule.

CMS noted that we should have discussed in our conclusions the implications of omitting "shared services" providers from our analysis, as these providers tend to have higher costs. As we discussed in the report, ambulance providers that could not separately report the costs of the ambulance portion of their business were excluded because their cost data were determined to be unreliable. Consequently, we have no basis or information to suggest that providers with shared services have higher or lower ccsts than other providers.

Ambulance industry associations generally agreed with our findings. However, the associations raised various concerns regarding our calculations and assumptions. Two associations questioned the inclusion in our analysis of ambulance providers that used unpaid staff and suggested that it might have been more appropriate to focus on providers who bear the full cost of providing ambulance services. As we note in the report, use of unpaid staff by ambulance providers is widespread with an estimated two-fifths of the industry relying substantially on volunteers in 2004. Thus, in order for our analysis to be representative of ambulance providers, we included those that used volunteer staff. We recognize that use of volunteer staff affects ambulance providers' costs and included the percentage of volunteer hours as a control variable in our cost model.

Two associations were concerned that we did not allow for the effect of Medicare bad debt in our analysis and may have therefore overestimated payments. We acknowledge that bad debt will affect the percentage of costs recoverable for providing ambulance services. However, we explicitly state that our payment estimates assume providers are paid the full Medicare payment amounts. It was beyond the scope of our study to estimate the effect of Medicare bad debt on ambulance payments or to determine the extent to which payments should be adjusted to reflect bad debt.

Two associations expressed concern that our analysis showed a 3 percent increase in payments to ambulance providers with the transition from the historical payment system to the fully implemented national fee schedule and thought payments should have been relatively level. We note that our analysis incorporated increases in mileage rates over time that likely accounted for some of this increase. In addition, when simulating payments under the national fee schedule, we assumed that providers would bill Medicare for all services they were entitled to bill. However, as we noted in the report, nearly half of the industry indicated that a state or local government approves the fees they may charge, and some providers are required to bill Medicare less than the allowed amount and therefore do not receive the maximum Medicare payment allowed under the fee schedule. This discrepancy between the state or local allowed amount and the actual Medicare payment could also account for some of the 3 percent increase.

CMS and the associations also provided technical comments and clarifications, which we incorporated as appropriate.

We are sending copies of this chapter to other interested congressional committees and the Administrator of CMS. We will also provide copies to others upon request. The report will also be available at no charge on the GAO Web site at http://www.gao.gov.

If you or your staff have any questions, please contact me at (202) 512-7119 or kingk@gao.gov. Contact points for our Offices of Congressional Relations and Public Affairs may be found on the last page of this chapter. GAO staff who made major contributions to this chapter are listed in appendix III.

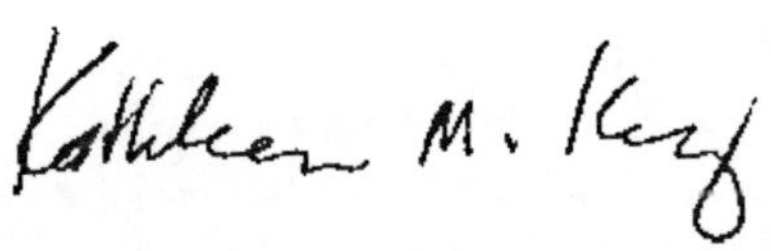

Kathleen M. King
Director, Health Care

Appendix I. Data and Methods

This appendix describes, in detail, the data and methods we used to respond to our research objectives and evaluate ambulance providers' costs per transport and Medicare payments under the national ambulance fee schedule. We conducted a survey of ambulance costs to collect cost data. We relied on these survey data for much of our analyses of costs and supplemented our survey results with information from other sources, including Medicare claims data, as appropriate. We also analyzed Medicare claims data to determine the effect of the national fee schedule and the Medicare Prescription Drug, Improvement and Modernization Act of 2003 (MMA) temporary payment provisions on payments, as well as to describe changes in beneficiaries' use of ambulance transports over time. We tested the internal consistency and reliability of the data from our survey and other non-Medicare data sources and determined that all data sources were adequate for our purposes. We conducted our work from July 2004 through April 2007 in accordance with generally accepted government auditing standards.

National Survey of Ground Ambulance Providers' Costs

To collect data on ground ambulance providers' costs, revenues, transports, and organizational characteristics for their most recently completed fiscal year, we mailed a survey to a nationally representative sample of 500 eligible ambulance service providers that billed Medicare in 2003.[41] We used a two-stage sampling process to select a stratified,[42] random sample of providers. In the first stage, we selected a preliminary sample of hospital and nonhospital-based providers for screening. In the second stage, we conducted telephone screening interviews to confirm eligibility for the study and, for nonhospital-based providers, to identify provider type. We obtained 321 completed surveys for a response rate of 64 percent. We excluded two cost outliers. We also excluded from our analysis providers that reported sharing ambulance costs with other institutions or other nonambulance services, including, but not limited to, all fire departments, after preliminary analysis revealed problems with the reliability of their reported costs. The resulting sample size was 215 providers. The results from our analysis are nationally representative of all Medicare ambulance providers that can distinguish their costs for providing ambulance services from the costs of other services they provide.[43] However, the small sample size and the variability of reported costs reduce the precision of our estimates.

Survey Instrument Development

To develop our survey instrument, we reviewed other survey instruments and analyses of ambulance cost data, consulted with experts in survey methods and the ambulance industry, and tested our survey instrument. We reviewed cost data collected in 1999 by Project HOPE Center for Health Affairs, which was a nonprofit health policy research organization, during a survey effort sponsored by the American Ambulance Association. We also reviewed other surveys of emergency medical services, as well as industry and association guidelines about emergency medical and ambulance services. In addition to surveying ambulance providers on their costs and revenues, we included questions to identify organizational and local area characteristics that might affect ambulance costs, such as the number of emergency transports and number of volunteer hours.

Industry experts and a survey specialist reviewed and commented on the draft survey instrument. We conducted a pilot test of the survey with 104 ambulance service providers as well. We redesigned and refined the instrument based on the experience of the pilot test. Then, to further refine the wording of our survey questions, we asked four types of ambulance service organizations and a former volunteer fire chief to pretest the instrument and point out any issues they noted. These pretests were conducted mostly by telephone—one pretest was in person.

Sample Design

We developed separate lists for all hospital-based and nonhospital-based providers from information maintained by the Centers for Medicare & Medicaid Services (CMS), the agency that oversees the Medicare program. Next, we used a two-stage sampling process to select a stratified, random sample of providers. In the first stage, we sorted each list by census division and predominant service area (urban, rural, or super-rural), began sampling the list at a random starting point, and chose providers at regular intervals from their respective lists. This method of sampling implicitly included representation across census divisions and service areas. In the second stage, telephone screening interviews were conducted with each sampled provider to confirm eligibility for the study and, for nonhospital-based providers, to identify their type—volunteer, fire department, government, or freestanding. Once a provider's type was established, providers were stratified by type and randomly selected to ensure somewhat equal representation among all provider types. We developed initial sample rates for each type of provider and adjusted the rates midway through the screening process. Each provider representative was told at the close of the telephone screening call whether the provider had been selected to participate in our survey. Finally, a survey instrument was mailed to the selected providers.

To identify nonhospital-based ambulance providers that billed Medicare, we contacted Medicare carriers[44] for a list of ambulance providers and matched this list to 2003 carrier claims for ambulance services by provider identification numbers. Our nonhospital-based sample frame included 12,082 unique provider identification numbers.[45] We later learned that a number of provider identification numbers in the nonhospital-based sample frame were duplicate entries for ambulance providers that had more than one Medicare provider identification number for the same location.[46] We analyzed the extent of duplication in the sample frame and reduced the estimated population size to 7,968. Although our sample frame included a substantial number of duplicate entries, there were only 28 duplicates among our first-stage sample of 900 nonhospital-based providers. The sample weights were adjusted to account for the duplicate entries in the sample frame.

To identify the total number of hospital-based ambulance providers that billed Medicare, we matched Medicare's Provider of Service file with Medicare Part A inpatient and outpatient claims for ambulance services. We excluded skilled nursing facilities for a total of 828 hospital-based ambulance service providers. We then selected a first-stage sample of 150 hospital-based ambulance providers.

To make our survey sample representative of all Medicare ambulance providers, the population from which the sample was drawn, we computed a sample weight for each respondent provider. The computation of the sample weight took into account the type of provider, sample rate, and the response rate for the type of provider—hospital, volunteer, fire department, government, or freestanding.

Survey Administration

We contracted with CODA Inc., an independent survey research firm, to perform the telephone screening and administer the mailed survey instrument.[47] The contractor screened the 900 nonhospital-based and 150 hospital-based providers we selected for our first-stage sample, and mailed the survey instrument to 500 eligible organizations, randomly sampled by provider type. In order to properly select our sample with even representation across all types of providers nationally, we designed our sampling strata using data collected from our pilot test.

CODA Inc., administered the mailed surveys and conducted all follow-up and data coding in coordination with us. Our survey period began in April 2005 and ran through September 2005. The survey instruments were mailed using Federal Express and 2-day Priority Mail. Telephone contact was initiated 3 business days after the instrument was mailed to ascertain when the respondent could return the completed instrument. Prompting and follow-up requests for data were conducted by phone and occurred whenever providers' returned instruments were incomplete, vague, or included conflicting responses to key items. In some cases, follow-up requests involved multiple contacts, faxing survey instruments, and spending an hour or more on the phone with the respondent. On average, more than 4 phone calls were made for each respondent with as many as 20 calls made to one respondent.

All requests for data were conducted by CODA Inc. staff following strict protocols that we developed. Respondents were encouraged to contact CODA Inc. and GAO via toll-free numbers, so that any questions or problems could be resolved. All survey data were double-key entered into an electronic file, and computer programs were checked for keying discrepancies and data inconsistencies. In all, we received 321 completed surveys; this represents a response rate of 64 percent.

Survey Data Validity and Reliability

In addition to the survey administration procedures described above, we took several measures to ensure that the data reported on the survey were valid and reliable.[48] First, the survey instrument included items intended to validate the reported cost data. We also used strict protocols during follow-up to validate the reported cost data. For example, if respondents could not provide cost breakdowns by the categories listed in our survey instrument, a separate phone protocol was used to verify the reported cost data.

Second, we tested the data for internal consistency and excluded cases when necessary. Computer analyses were performed to identify and, where possible, correct any inconsistencies in responses or other errors. We also excluded 2 providers that appeared to be cost outliers. These providers had costs per transport that were at least three standard deviations above the mean of the standard statistical distribution (the lognormal), and no other variables explained their extraordinary costs. Through our analyses, we determined that the costs reported by providers that shared costs with other institutions or offered other services appeared to be unreliable. We found the costs reported by these "shared costs" providers to be highly variable, which may reflect inconsistent methods for separating staff time and other resources across different services. Therefore, we excluded these providers—including but not limited to all fire departments—from our analysis. The resulting sample size was 215 providers, representing a population of more than 5,200 providers without shared costs.[49]

Third, we compared information reported on the survey to information on Medicare claims submitted by respondents, such as the number of Medicare transports and percentage of emergency Medicare transports. All computer syntax was peer reviewed and verified by separate programmers to ensure that the syntax was written and executed correctly.

We used providers' total costs and total transports reported on the survey to compute providers' average costs per transport. This cost information and other information about revenues and provider characteristics were used to model ambulance costs per transport. Although these survey data were self-reported and had not been audited, based on efforts to validate the data, computer testing, and corrections and comparisons with Medicare data, we have concluded that they were sufficiently valid and reliable for our purposes.

Interpretation of Confidence Intervals and Analysis of Nonrespondents

All sample surveys are subject to sampling error—that is, the extent to which the survey results differ from what would have been obtained if we had collected responses from every ambulance provider in the country. Because we used a sample, it is only one of a large number of samples that we might have drawn. As each sample could have provided different estimates, we express our confidence in the precision of our particular sample's results as a 95 percent confidence interval.[50] This is the interval that would contain the actual value for all providers for 95 percent of the samples we could have drawn. As a result, we are 95 percent confident that the reported confidence intervals based on the mailed survey include the true values for all providers. For this reason, all costs per transport and provider margins are reported with their confidence intervals.

We also analyzed 2004 Medicare claims data for survey nonrespondents and compared this information with similar claims information for providers without shared costs in our sample. Nonrespondents served predominantly urban areas rather than rural or super-rural areas. On average, nonrespondents completed about half the number of Medicare transports in 2004 compared with providers without shared costs. Nonrespondents also had a higher percentage of basic life support (BLS) transports, as opposed to advanced life support (ALS) and more complex transports, and about the same percentage of nonemergency transports compared with providers without shared costs.

It is unclear whether nonrespondents had higher or lower costs, on average, than providers without shared costs. In our regression analysis of the cost information for providers without shared costs, we found that those with fewer transports per year generally had higher costs per transport than those with more transports. Providers without shared costs that served predominately urban areas had lower costs compared with providers serving super-rural areas. We also found that providers with higher percentages of BLS transports had lower costs compared to providers with no BLS transports. Although nonrespondents' characteristics differed from those of providers without shared costs, these differences were associated with both higher and lower costs among providers without shared costs. Therefore, we have no basis for concluding that nonresponse has biased our cost estimates in any particular direction.

Table 8. Provider and Local Area Characteristics Included in Analysis of Average Cost per Transport, 2004

Characteristic	Measure	Source of data
Transport volume	Indicator of volume group: <=2,000, 2001-3000, 3001-4,000, 4001-5000, 5001-6000, 6001+	GAO Survey of Ambulance Services
Type of provider	Staffing and organizational structure	GAO Survey of Ambulance Services
Productivity	Transports per staffed ambulance hour[a]	GAO Survey of Ambulance Services
Price of fuel	Annualized average retail price of fuel in the provider's zip code	Oil Price Information Service
Building rent	Price per square foot of office space in the provider's zip code	United States Postal Service
Cost of labor used by providers	Geographic practice cost index (GPCI)[b]	Medicare Ambulance Fee Schedule Public Use File
	Percentage of volunteer hours, including on-call time	GAO Survey of Ambulance Services
Revenue derived from local tax support	Community tax support as a percentage of total ambulance provider revenue[c]	GAO Survey of Ambulance Services
Regulation of fees	State or local government approval of fees charged	GAO Survey of Ambulance Services
Mix and intensity of transports	Percentage of emergency transports	GAO Survey of Ambulance Services
	Percentage of Medicare transports that are BLS	Medicare claims
Service area	Percentage of Medicare transports that are rural	Medicare claims
	Percentage of Medicare transports that are super-rural	Medicare claims
Census division in which the ambulance provider was located	Census Division 1 – New England	Medicare claims
	Census Division 2 – Middle Atlantic	Medicare claims
	Census Division 3 – East North Central	Medicare claims
	Census Division 4 – West North Central	Medicare claims
	Census Division 5 – South Atlantic	Medicare claims
	Census Division 6 – East South Central	Medicare claims
	Census Division 7 – West South Central	Medicare claims
	Census Division 8 – Mountain	Medicare claims
	Census Division 9 – Pacific	Medicare claims

Sources: 2005 GAO Survey of Ambulance Services, Oil Price Information Service, United States Postal Service, Medicare Ambulance Fee Schedule Public Use File, and Medicare claims.

[a] This measure was computed as the total number of transports in the year divided by the total number of hours that an ambulance and crew were staffed and available

to respond to an emergency call. This measure is also known as unit hours of utilization.

[b] The practice expense portion of the physician fee schedule's GPCI is used to adjust the ambulance national fee schedule.

[c] This measure was computed as the total amount of revenues derived from community tax support divided by total revenues.

Modeling Ambulance Costs per Transport

We analyzed the relationship between providers' average costs of ambulance transports and the provider and local area characteristics that may have affected their average costs. We used regression analysis to examine the effect of these characteristics on providers' costs per transport. We then used the results from this regression analysis to predict the average costs per transport across all providers without shared costs, based on five key provider characteristics: (1) total transports per year, (2) percentage of BLS Medicare transports, (3) percentage of Medicare transports in rural and super-rural areas, (4) number of ambulance transports per staffed hour, and (5) amount of revenue derived from local tax support.

To perform these analyses, we identified measures and data sources for each of the provider and local area characteristics that we identified as potentially contributing to differences in costs per transport. A summary of these characteristics, measures we used to assess their potential relationship to costs per transport, and data sources used is presented in table 8.

Average Cost Regression Analysis—Methods and Results

Our regression analysis modeled the average cost of a transport at the provider level as a function of the provider and local area characteristics described above. We modeled the lognormal distribution of average cost per transport for a provider, which was calculated as the log of total costs divided by the total number of transports for that provider. We estimated the model using least squares[51] and applied the appropriate sample weights. We used the statistical program SUDAAN® in SAS to estimate this model, which takes account of the sample stratification and weighting to obtain appropriate parameter estimates and standard errors. We tested for and found no specification problems in the model resulting from heteroscedasticity, misspecification, or evidence of a particular observation having undue influence.

Table 9. Results for Average Cost of an Ambulance Transport Regression—Estimated Effects of Selected Provider and Local Area Characteristics on the Average Cost of Ambulance Transports for Providers, Not Including Impact of Productivity and Community Tax Support

Characteristic	Variable used to measure characteristic	Parameter estimate	t-value
Transport volume[a]	2,001-3,000 per year	-0.18	-1.70*
	3,001-4,000 per year	-0.35	2.98***
	4,001-5,000 per year	-0.34	3.33***
	5,001-6,000 per year	-0.52	2.71***
	6,001 + per year	-0.34	2.86***
Cost of labor used by providers	GPCI	1.34	2.27**
	Percentage of volunteer hours, including on-call time	-0.28	2.73***
Regulation of fees	State or local government approval of fees charged	-0.08	-1.00
Mix and intensity of transports	Percentage of emergency transports	0.17	0.99
	Percentage of Medicare transports that are BLS	-0.28	-2.39**
Service area[b]	Percentage of Medicare transports that are rural	0.16	1.61
	Percentage of Medicare transports that are super-rural	0.42	3.11***
Census division in which the ambulance provider was located[c]	Census Division 1 – New England	-0.27	-1.66*
	Census Division 2 – Middle Atlantic	-0.24	-1.66*
	Census Division 3 – East North Central	0.23	1.61
	Census Division 5 – South Atlantic	0.07	0.41
	Census Division 6 – East South Central	-0.07	-0.43
	Census Division 7 – West South Central	-0.16	-0.85
	Census Division 8 – Mountain	0.15	0.97
	Census Division 9 – Pacific	-0.27	-1.39
	Intercept	4.83	8.73***
	R-squared	0.33	
	Observations	205	

Sources: GAO analysis of 2005 GAO Survey of Ambulance Services, Medicare Ambulance Fee Schedule Public Use File, and Medicare claims.

*** significant at the 1 percent level.

** significant at the 5 percent level.

* significant at the 10 percent level.

[a] Transports less than or equal to 2,000 per year is the excluded category. In order for the regression model's parameters to be estimated, we needed to exclude one of the transport volume categories.

[b] The percentage of Medicare transports that are urban was the excluded category. In order for the regression model's parameters to be estimated, we needed to exclude one of the service area categories.

[c] The West North Central census division was the excluded category. In order for the regression model's parameters to be estimated, we needed to exclude one of the census divisions.

Table 10. Results for Average Cost of an Ambulance Transport Regression—Estimated Effects of Selected Provider and Local Area Characteristics on the Average Cost of Ambulance Transports for Providers, Including Impact of Productivity and Community Tax Support

Characteristic	Variable used to measure characteristic	Parameter estimate	t-value
Transport volume[a]	2,001 -3,000 per year	-0.17	-1.84*
	3,001-4,000 per year	-0.30	-2.69***
	4,001-5,000 per year	-0.34	-3.40***
	5,001-6,000 per year	-0.31	-1.72*
	6,001+ per year	-0.22	-1.92*
Cost of labor used by providers	GPCI	1.29	2.62***
	Percentage of volunteer hours, including on-call time	-0.10	-0.79
Regulation of fees	State or local government approval of fees charged	-0.11	-1.49
Mix and intensity of transports	Percentage of emergency transports	0.06	0.29
	Percentage of Medicare transports that are BLS	-0.31	-2.25**
Service area[b]	Percentage of Medicare transports that are rural	0.06	0.67
	Percentage of Medicare transports that are super-rural	0.26	1.93*
Productivity	Transports per staffed ambulance hour	-0.24	-2.76***
Community tax support	Community tax support as a percentage of total ambulance provider revenue	0.59	3.81***
Census division in which the ambulance provider was located[c]	Census Division 1 – New England	-0.24	-1.55
	Census Division 2 – Middle Atlantic	-0.24	-1.42
	Census Division 3 – East North Central	0.17	1.04
	Census Division 5 – South Atlantic	0.09	0.48
	Census Division 6 – East South Central	-0.16	-1.00
	Census Division 7 – West South Central	-0.30	-1.48

	Census Division 8 – Mountain	0.20	1.38
	Census Division 9 – Pacific	0.02	0.12
	Intercept	4.95	9.81***
	R-squared	0.51	
	Observations	157	

Sources: GAO analysis of 2005 GAO Survey of Ambulance Services, Medicare Ambulance Fee Schedule Public Use File, and Medicare claims.

*** significant at the 1 percent level.

** significant at the 5 percent level.

* significant at the 10 percent level.

[a] Transports less than or equal to 2,000 per year is the excluded category. In order for the regression model's parameters to be estimated, we needed to exclude one of the transport volume categories.

[b] The percentage of Medicare transports that are urban was the excluded category. In order for the regression model's parameters to be estimated, we needed to exclude one of the service area categories.

[c] The West North Central census division was the excluded category. In order for the regression model's parameters to be estimated, we needed to exclude one of the census divisions.

Tables 9 and 10 show the regression results for estimating the determinants of cost per transport. We ran two sets of average cost regressions. The first regression results, in table 9, do not include two provider characteristics, (1) transports per staffed ambulance hour and (2) community tax support as a percentage of total ambulance provider revenue, because data on these variables were not available for a number of providers in our sample. Including these variables as explanatory independent variables reduces the number of observations in the regression from 205 to 157. Nevertheless, we wanted to measure the impact of these policy variables, in addition to maintaining a larger sample size, in order to have a more precise estimate of the impact of the other explanatory variables. Therefore, we ran the same regression model with and without these two explanatory variables.

We estimated the average cost per transport associated with a range of values for each of five provider characteristics by using our regression result parameter estimates and fixed values for five provider characteristics. For each of the five provider characteristics, we assumed that all providers in the sample had the same value for one provider characteristic and used the national average value for all other characteristics. The five provider characteristics of interest were (1) total transports per year, (2) percentage of BLS Medicare transports, percentage of Medicare transports in rural and super-rural areas, number of transports per staffed ambulance hour, and (5) amount of revenue derived from local tax support. We estimated the cost per transport associated with two or more values for each of five provider characteristics. Our estimates are presented in table 2 of this chapter.

In order to create the estimated costs per transport for one value of a provider characteristic, we performed the following steps. First, we modified the data set we used in the regression model by assigning one fixed value for one provider characteristic, such as the percentage of super-rural Medicare transports, for all observations in the data set. For this characteristic, we fixed the percentage of Medicare super-rural transports to 100 percent and the percentage of Medicare rural transports to 0 percent for all observations in the data set.52 Second, we used our regression result parameter estimates for all the other characteristics in the regression model and calculated an estimated average cost per transport for each provider. Third, we computed the mean of these estimated costs per transport. We report this hypothetical value as the estimated average cost per transport associated with the fixed value of the provider characteristic of interest. In the example above, we computed our estimated average cost per transport of a super-rural Medicare transport assuming that every provider in the sample provided only super- rural Medicare transports and their other characteristics—volume and mix of transports, productivity, and amount of local tax support—were the national average.

Estimating Average Medicare Ambulance Payments and Use of Transports with Claims Data

To assess the effect of the ambulance national fee schedule on Medicare payments, we used Medicare claims data to compute average payments in 2001, before the implementation of the fee schedule, and in 2004, 2 years after the phase-in of the national fee schedule had begun. For all analyses of Medicare payments, we expressed payments in 2004 dollars. We also used Medicare claims data and payment formulas as specified in federal regulations to simulate average payments under the national fee schedule in 2010, after all the MMA provisions are due to expire on December 31, 2009, but computed these payments in 2004 dollars, the year that best reflects the cost data collected in our survey. We used the simulated payments to compute providers' Medicare margins, a comparison that assumes that providers' cost structures under the fee schedule would be the same as they were in 2004.53 We also assessed the effect of the MMA temporary payment provisions on payments in 2004 using Medicare claims data by examining the change in payments from the first half of the year, before the MMA changes were implemented, with the second half of the year, when MMA payment provisions had their maximum effect.

Table 11. Census Divisions

Census divisions	States
New England	Connecticut, Maine, Massachusetts, New Hampshire, Rhode Island, Vermont
Middle Atlantic	New Jersey, New York, Pennsylvania
East North Central	Illinois, Indiana, Michigan, Ohio, Wisconsin
West North Central	Iowa, Kansas, Minnesota, Missouri, Nebraska, North Dakota, South Dakota
South Atlantic	Delaware, District of Columbia, Florida, Georgia, Maryland, North Carolina, South Carolina, Virginia, West Virginia
East South Central	Alabama, Kentucky, Mississippi, Tennessee
West South Central	Arkansas, Louisiana, Oklahoma, Texas
Mountain	Arizona, Colorado, Idaho, Montana, Nevada, New Mexico, Utah, Wyoming
Pacific	Alaska, California, Hawaii, Oregon, Washington

Source: U.S. Census Bureau.

To estimate average Medicare ambulance payments in 2001 and 2004, we used Medicare Part A and Part B claims data from Medicare's National Claims History files. We constructed summary data sets with the number of ambulance transports, miles, and their Medicare payments, total[54] and by level of service,[55] at the zip code level for 2001 and 2004 to compare payments over time. These data sets were classified by three geographic levels: national; census divisions; and urban, rural, and super-rural areas.

Census divisions were categorized according to the U.S. Census Bureau's guidelines. (See table 11 for a listing of census divisions.) CMS designates urban, rural, and super-rural areas according to population density.

Medicare Payment Calculations and Simulation

We chose to examine payments in three distinct time periods: 2001, the first half of 2004, and the second half of 2004. The year before the national fee schedule was implemented was 2001. The first half of 2004 represented a period after the implementation of the national fee schedule but before the introduction of MMA temporary payment changes. It also coincided with the year for which we have cost data. The second half of 2004 represented a period after the introduction of MMA provisions when the regional fee schedule had its greatest effect.

In general, average Medicare payments were estimated as the sum of the average base rate payment—that is, the amount paid for the level of service56—and the average mileage payment. Base rate payments and mileage payments for each period were computed separately. Average Medicare payments were calculated nationally; by census division; and by urban, rural, and super-rural areas. All payments are expressed in 2004 dollars.

For the first half of 2004, the average base rate payment was calculated by dividing total base rate payments by the total number of transports provided in the first half of 2004. For 2001 and the second half of 2004, the average service-level base payment rate was calculated by dividing total base rate payments for each level of service by the total number of transports provided at each level of service. Then we computed a weighted average base rate payment for 2001 and for the second half of 2004 by applying the percentage of transports for each level of service (also known as the mix of services) for the first half of 2004 to the service- level base payment rates in 2001 and the second half of 2004, respectively. The 2001 payments were adjusted to 2004 dollars by multiplying weighted average base rate payment by the ratio of the 2004 Consumer Price Index for All Urban Consumers (CPI-U) over the 2001 CPI-U.

For simulated 2010 base rate payments, we multiplied the 2004 conversion factor (CF) and applicable relative value unit (RVU) for each level of service to compute the service level payments.57 Then, we computed a weighted average base rate payment by applying the service mix from the first half of 2004 to the 2004 service-level payments. The weighted average base-rate payment was adjusted for regional differences in the cost of providing ambulance services by the GPCI.58 In accordance with CMS's payment methodology, only 70 percent of the average base rate payment was adjusted by the GPCI.

Average mileage payments were calculated by multiplying the average miles per transport in each geographic level from the first half of 2004 by mileage rates in the other periods. (See tables 12 and 13.) For example, when estimating average 2001 mileage payments for urban transports, the 2001 mileage rate applicable to urban areas was used,59 but the average mile per transport in urban areas for the first half of 2004 was applied. For simulated payments in 2010, mileage rates from the first half of 2004 were applied. For average national and census division mileage payments, weighted mileage rates were applied reflecting the applicable percentage of urban and rural miles in the first half of 2004. Because the average mile per transport for super-rural areas was above 17, simulated payments for super-rural areas were computed using the two rural mileage rates—$8.48 for miles 1 through 17 and $5.65 for miles 18 through 50.

Analysis of Medicare Margins

We used simulated Medicare payments and costs per transport to compute Medicare margins under the national fee schedule after MMA temporary payment provisions are due to expire, to determine how much providers stood to lose or gain. To do this, we merged the survey results with providers' Medicare payment information from 2004. For each provider, we computed the mix of services and the average miles per transport for January 2004 through June 2004. This information was used to simulate each provider's average Medicare payment under the national fee schedule in 2010 after all MMA temporary payment provisions are set to expire on December 31, 2009.60 We subtracted the provider's 2004 cost per transport from the simulated average Medicare payment under the national fee schedule, and then divided by the simulated average payment to compute the provider's Medicare margin.

Estimating Use of Ambulance Transports by Medicare Beneficiaries

To estimate transports per 1,000 Medicare beneficiaries, we supplemented our Medicare claims data with CMS enrollment data from 2001 and 2004, which contained information regarding Medicare beneficiaries. The numbers of Medicare beneficiaries in 2001 and 2004 were measured as the number of months beneficiaries were covered by Medicare in each year divided by 12. A ratio of the number of transports over the number of Medicare beneficiaries was estimated in each year and multiplied by 1,000.

Table 12. Average Mile per Transport, First Half of 2004

Area	Average mile per transport
National	9
Urban	7
Rural	13
Super-rural	20
East North Central	9
East South Central	12
Middle Atlantic	7
Mountain	9
Pacific	7
New England	7
South Atlantic	10
West North Central	14
West South Central	11

Source: 2004 Medicare claims.

Table 13. Mileage Rates

Period	Urban	Rural (1-17)	Rural (18-50)
2001	$5.33	$5.33	$5.33
1/1/04 – 6/30/04	5.65	8.48	5.65
7/31/04 – 12/31/04	5.71	8.65	5.76
Simulated fee schedule	5.65	8.48	5.65

Sources: 67 *Fed. Reg.* 9100 and 2004 Medicare Ambulance Fee Schedule Public Use File.

Notes: All mileage rates are expressed in 2004 dollars. The 2001 mileage rate is based on the mileage rate for ground ambulance services used by CMS when creating the national fee schedule. Rural mileage rates also apply to super-rural transports.

Medicare Claims Data Reliability

Medicare claims data, which are used by the Medicare program as a record of payments made to health care providers, are closely monitored by both CMS and Medicare carriers—contractors that process, review, and pay claims for Medicare Part B-covered services, including ambulance services. The data are subject to various internal controls, including checks and edits performed by the carriers before claims are submitted to CMS for payment approval. Although we did not review these internal controls, we found the data to be sufficiently reliable for the purposes of this chapter. We also assessed the reliability of CMS's enrollment data. We found these data to be sufficiently reliable for the purposes of this chapter.

APPENDIX II. COMMENTS FROM THE CENTERS FOR MEDICARE & MEDICAID SERVICES

DEPARTMENT OF HEALTH & HUMAN SERVICES — Centers for Medicare & Medicaid Services

Administrator
Washington, DC 20201

DATE: [illegible] 2007

TO: Kathleen M. King
Director, Health Care
Government Accountability Office

FROM: Leslie V. Norwalk, Esq.
Acting Administrator

SUBJECT: Government Accountability Office (GAO) Draft Report: "AMBULANCE PROVIDERS: Costs and Expected Medicare Margins Vary Greatly" (GAO-07-383)

The Centers for Medicare & Medicaid Services (CMS) appreciates the opportunity to review and provide comments on the GAO draft report entitled "AMBULANCE PROVIDERS: Costs and Expected Medicare Margins Vary Greatly." On April 1, 2002, CMS implemented the Medicare ambulance fee schedule with a 5-year transition period. The fee schedule was established through a negotiated rulemaking process, as required by the statute, which allowed interested stakeholders to participate in its development. During the transition period, Congress enacted several temporary ambulance provisions in the Medicare Modernization Act of 2003, including bonus payments for ambulance services in rural pick-up areas. All of these legislative provisions will sunset by December 31, 2009. Since the ambulance fee schedule is a departure in payment structure from the prior methods of payment for ambulance services, GAO examined how ambulance companies were faring under the ambulance fee schedule and whether or not they have been successful and will be successful in the future in recovering their costs for services provided to Medicare beneficiaries under the ambulance fee schedule.

We appreciate the effort that GAO has put into this report and, for the most part, the report reinforces CMS' own findings. Generally, ambulance services incur a cost of readiness, which was built into the ambulance fee schedule payment structure, and rural ambulance companies incur higher costs per trip than urban ambulance companies due to a lower expected volume of trips provided to the Medicare population.

GAO Recommendation:

CMS should monitor utilization of ambulance transports to ensure that Medicare payments are adequate to provide for beneficiary access to ambulance services, particularly in super-rural areas.

CMS Response:

We agree with GAO's recommendation. In fact, we stated in the 2006 final rule (71 FR 69717) published on December 1, 2006, that we would continue to monitor all ambulance rates and would make adjustments should the original assumptions that we made during the development of the ambulance fee schedule prove to need adjustment. Further, in this same final rule (71 FR 69714), we implemented use of the Rural Urban Commuting Areas (RUCAs) in conjunction with recognizing the 2000 decennial census population data. The RUCAs allow us to recognize levels of rurality in every zip code across the country. Since ambulance payments under Medicare are based on the point of pick-up, the level of detail provided by the use of the RUCAs is of particular benefit to rural areas within urban counties, allowing these zip code locations to receive the benefit of the higher rural payments under the ambulance fee schedule.

We note that many of the ambulance providers with "shared services" that were omitted from the analysis have higher than average costs. These include hospital-based providers and joint fire/ambulance services. We recommend that the GAO review the survey data and other data sources from prior studies for these groups. GAO should discuss the implications of omitting these groups in the concluding section of the report.

In conclusion, we deeply appreciate GAO's efforts in examining these important issues. We look forward to working with you in the future as we monitor ambulance services under the ambulance fee schedule. As we stated in the final rule on December 1, 2006, we are committed to continuing to monitor these issues to ensure that the ambulance fee schedule accurately reflects the realities of services provided to Medicare beneficiaries by the ambulance industry.

Attachment

Related GAO Products

Ambulance Services: Medicare Payments Can Be Better Targeted to Trips in Less Densely Populated Rural Areas. GAO-03-986. Washington, D.C.: September 19, 2003.

Ambulance Services: Changes Needed to Improve Medicare Payment Policies and Coverage Decisions. GAO-02-244T. Washington, D.C.: November 15, 2001.

Emergency Medical Services: Reported Needs Are Wide-Ranging, With A Growing Focus on Lack of Data. GAO-02-28. Washington, D.C.: October 12, 2001.

Rural Ambulances: Medicare Fee Schedule Payments Could Be Better Targeted. GAO/HEHS-00-115. Washington, D.C.: July 17, 2000.

End Notes

[1] We use the term providers to refer to all types of organizations that provide ambulance transports for Medicare beneficiaries.

[2] 42 U.S.C. § 1395m(l).

[3] Reasonable-cost payments were based on the provider's cost of providing ambulance services as reported on cost reports.

[4] Reasonable-charge payments were based on the bill from the ambulance service provider but were subject to an upper limit.

[5] The national fee schedule applies to ground and air ambulance services, but this chapter and our analysis are limited to ground ambulance services only, which include water ambulance services and account for nearly all ambulance services. We use the terms service, transport, and ambulance service to refer to ground ambulance transport services only.

[6] Pub. L. No. 108-173, § 414, 117 Stat. 2066, 2278-80 (2003).

[7] Pub. L. No. 106-554, appendix F, § 436, 114 Stat. 2763, 2763A-527 (2000).

[8] The GAO Survey of Ambulance Services asked providers to report on their organizations' costs of providing ground ambulance services. As such, the survey measures organizations' expenses, or spending, for ground ambulance services.

[9] The sample was stratified by five types of ambulance providers: hospital-based, volunteer, fire-based, government, and freestanding.

[10] To make our survey sample representative of all Medicare ambulance providers, we computed a sample weight for each respondent provider.

[11] We applied our sample weights to the subgroup so the providers were nationally representative of all ambulance service providers without shared costs.

[12] To define urban, rural, and super-rural transports, CMS uses the metropolitan statistical areas (MSA) definitions established by the Office of Management and Budget. During the period of our study, CMS defined urban transports as those that originate within MSAs and New England county metropolitan areas (NECMA), rural transports as those that originate in rural counties that are outside of MSAs and NECMAs as well as small towns and rural areas within MSAs or NECMAs that are isolated from central areas by distance or other features, such as mountains. CMS defines super-rural transports as those that originate in the bottom 25 percent of rural areas as defined by population density.

[13] This comparison assumes that providers' cost structures under the fee schedule would be the same as they were in 2004.

[14] The Commission on Accreditation of Ambulance Services and the Commission of Accreditation of Medical Transport Systems have established ambulance service accreditation standards.

[15] The National Association of State EMS Officials has worked with other industry associations and federal partners to develop tools for measuring the performance of EMS systems: (1) EMS system indicators, which were released for public comment and are being finalized; (2) the National EMS Information Management System; and (3) a cost framework for cost analysis in EMS research. The American Ambulance Association published its *Community Guide to Ensure High-Performance Emergency Ambulance Services* in 2004.

[16] Unless otherwise noted, all background information on the ambulance industry is from the GAO 2005 Survey of Ambulance Services. These estimates are based on the 321 total providers that responded to our survey.

[17] BLS services include basic, noninvasive interventions to reduce morbidity and mortality associated with acute out-of-hospital medical and traumatic emergencies.

[18] ALS services include advanced, invasive, and pharmacological interventions to reduce morbidity and mortality associated with acute out-of-hospital medical and traumatic emergencies.

[19] Under the Medicare program, there are seven levels of ambulance transports. BLS and ALS transports each constitute two levels, emergency or nonemergency. The remaining levels of service—ALS Level 2 and specialty care transport (both of which involve invasive or specialized care) and paramedic ALS intercept (when a paramedic provides ALS services but does not transport the patient)—made up less than 2 percent of all Medicare transports in 2004.

[20] EMT-Basic personnel are trained in BLS services only. EMT-Intermediate personnel are qualified to perform essential advanced techniques and to administer a limited number of medications. Paramedics have the competencies of EMT-Intermediate personnel in addition to other enhanced skills and can administer additional interventions and medications.

[21] Cross-trained staff typically refers to firefighters who are also trained as EMTs.

[22] We defined substantial use of volunteer staff as 20 percent or more of staff hours spent providing ambulance services, exclusive of administration.

[23] Rural areas can also be small towns and rural areas within large metropolitan counties that are isolated from central areas by distance or other features, such as mountains.

[24] From this point forward in the report, we refer to providers that served predominately urban, rural, and super-rural areas as urban, rural, and super-rural providers, respectively. We classified providers as super-rural if 60 percent or more of their Medicare transports in 2004 originated in a super-rural zip code. We classified providers as rural if they did not meet the super-rural definition and 60 percent or more of their Medicare transports in 2004 originated in rural or super-rural zip codes. We defined providers as urban if they did not meet the rural or super-rural classifications.

[25] A subscription program is an arrangement in which an ambulance service provider is paid an annual fee for providing emergency transportation for a community.

[26] In 2004, the annual spending of providers that responded to our survey ranged from less than $10,000 to more than $70 million.

[27] This estimate is based on a smaller sample of 209 providers that reported Medicare revenues and total revenues on the GAO 2005 Survey of Ambulance Services.

[28] Medicare ambulance transports must be deemed medically necessary in order for Medicare payments to be disbursed.

[29] There is an RVU for each of the seven levels of service defined by Medicare.

[30] The practice expense portion of the physician fee schedule's GPCI is used to adjust the ambulance national fee schedule.

[31] *See* 42 C.F.R. § 414.601 *et seq.*

[32] In this chapter we use the term regions to refer to the nine census divisions as defined by the U.S. Census Bureau. See table 11 in app. I for a description of the nine census divisions.

[33] The national fee schedule portion blend with historical payments includes mileage payments. The regional fee schedule is only applicable to the base rate payment.

[34] GAO, *Ambulance Services: Medicare Payments Can Be Better Targeted to Trips in Less Densely Populated Rural Areas*, GAO-03-986 (Washington, D.C.: Sept. 19, 2003).

[35] Transports per staffed hour is the total number of transports divided by the total number of hours that an ambulance and crew were staffed and available to respond to an emergency call.

[36] Because our cost information is estimated from a sample of providers, all costs per transport are reported with confidence intervals. The range of the confidence interval is affected by the variability of the responses within the sample and the size of the sample. See app. I for a full discussion of our sample, methods, and computations.

[37] The average cost per transport of super-rural providers without shared costs was based on the average costs of survey respondents without shared costs that served predominantly super-rural areas, and reflects the different characteristics of those respondents, including the volume of trips they provided. It is different from the estimated average cost of a super-rural transport based on our regression analysis.

[38] For each characteristic, we measured its effect on providers' average cost per transport, independent of other characteristics, by assuming the national average value for the other variables.

[39] GAO-03-986.

[40] The estimated average cost of a super-rural transport is different from the average cost per transport of super-rural providers without shared costs that was explained in footnote 37. The estimated average cost of a super-rural transport was calculated using regression analysis that assumed all providers without shared costs only performed super-rural transports and had the national average for the other variables in our analysis. See our app. I for more details on our methodology.

[41] Our survey asked providers to report on their organizations' costs of providing ground ambulance services.

[42] The sample was stratified by types of ambulance providers: hospital-based, volunteer, fire departments, government, and freestanding.

[43] Our cost analysis sample includes only those providers that could apportion the ground ambulance component of any cost shared between their ambulance services and other services. Thus, our results only reflect the experiences of providers that did not share costs or that could feasibly apportion them.

[44] Carriers are private companies that have contracts with Medicare to administer payment of providers' bills for covered Medicare Part B services.

[45] We excluded provider identification numbers that had been selected to participate in the pilot study.

[46] Duplicate entries for the same nonhospital provider were identified by name, address, and other information.

[47] CODA Inc. also administered the 1999 ambulance survey for Project HOPE and our pilot survey. During the course of the contract, CODA Inc. became Survey and Epidemiology Services Division of Social & Scientific Systems, Inc.

[48] For a randomly selected subsample of 30 providers—6 of each type of ambulance provider—we requested providers' financial records to match to their survey responses. We were only able to validate costs, revenues, and transport volumes for 2 providers in the subsample because providers either did not return supporting documentation or the categories—particularly those for costs—on providers' supporting documentation were different from those on the survey. As a result, we concluded that this method for validating survey data was not viable because of differences in data reporting, particularly cost categories, on providers' supporting documents.

[49] We could not determine a separate response rate for our subgroup of providers without shared costs because we could not identify which nonrespondents in our original sample were providers without shared costs. However, we have no reason to believe that the response rate for providers without shared costs would be different from the overall survey response rate.

[50] The range of the confidence interval is affected by the variability of the responses within the sample and the size of the sample.

[51] Least squares is a common method of regression analysis.

[52] The percentage of super-rural and rural Medicare transports were two separate variables in our model and the percentage of urban Medicare transports was our reference category. To assume that 100 percent of a provider's Medicare transports were rural, we set the percentage of rural Medicare transports to 100 percent and the percentage of super-rural Medicare transports to 0 percent. To assume that 100 percent of a provider's Medicare transports were urban, we set the percentage of super-rural Medicare transports to 0 percent and the percentage of rural Medicare transports to 0 percent.

[53] The Medicare margin reflects the percentage difference between the average Medicare payment and a provider's cost per transport. It was computed as the difference between the average Medicare payment and the cost per transport, divided by the payment.

[54] Total ambulance payments in 2001 and 2004 included any payments made for supplies in addition to mileage payments and service-level payments.

[55] Under the Medicare program, there are seven levels of ambulance transports. BLS and ALS transports each constitute two levels, emergency and nonemergency. The remaining levels of service are ALS Level 2 and specialty care transport (both of which involve invasive or specialized care) and paramedic ALS intercept (when a paramedic provides ALS services but does not transport the patient).

[56] Estimated average base rate payments for 2001 and 2004 included ambulance supply payments. Under the fee schedule, the base rate payment was meant to incorporate the transport and any necessary services or supplies used during the transport.

[57] Ambulance RVUs account for the relative resources needed to provide services during an ambulance transport. There is one RVU for each of the seven levels of service.

[58] In many cases, more than one GPCI would apply to our average base rate payment. For these cases we applied an average GPCI, which was weighted by the total number of transports in each geographic area of interest—national; census division; or urban, rural, or super-rural area.

[59] The 2001 mileage payments were eventually adjusted to 2004 dollars.

[60] We simulated the average payments under the national fee schedule in the same way described earlier in this appendix.

CHAPTER SOURCES

The following chapters have been previously published:

Chapter 1 – This is an edited, reformatted and augmented version of Congressional Research Service publication, Report RS22738, dated January 12, 2010.

Chapter 2 – This is an edited, reformatted and augmented version of United States Government Accountability Office publication GAO-09-347, dated April 2009.

Chapter 3 – This is an edited, reformatted and augmented version of Congressional Research Service publication, Report R40176, dated February 2, 2010.

Chapter 4 – This is an edited, reformatted and augmented version of Congressional Research Service publication, Report R40159, dated March 30, 2009.

Chapter 5 – This is an edited, reformatted and augmented version of United States Government Accountability Office publication GAO-07-383, dated May 2007

INDEX

E

F

G

H

I

Q

R

S

T

U

V

W